T0000294

Soberish

Kayla Lyons

Soberish

The
Science Based
Guide to Taking
Your Power Back
from Alcohol

WATKINS
Sharing Wisdom
Since 1893

Soberish
Kayla Lyons

First published in the UK and USA in 2023 by
Watkins, an imprint of Watkins Media Limited
Unit 11, Shepperton House, 83–93 Shepperton Road
London N1 3DF

enquiries@watkinspublishing.com

Design and typography copyright © Watkins Media Limited 2023
Text copyright © Kayla Lyons 2023

The right of Kayla Lyons to be identified as the Author of this text
has been asserted in accordance with the Copyright, Designs and
Patents Act of 1988.

All rights reserved. No part of this book may be reproduced in
any form or by any electronic or mechanical means, including
information storage and retrieval systems, without permission in
writing from the publisher, except by a reviewer who may quote brief
passages in a review.

Commissioning Editor: Lucy Carroll
Project Editor: Brittany Willis
Head of Design: Karen Smith
Design Concept: Alice Claire Coleman
Production: Uzma Taj

A CIP record for this book is available from the British Library
ISBN: 978-1-78678-752-1 (Paperback)
ISBN: 978-1-78678-760-6 (eBook)

10 9 8 7 6 5 4 3 2 1

Typeset by Lapiz
Printed in the United Kingdom by TJ Books Ltd

www.watkinspublishing.com

Publisher's note:
The information in this book is not a substitute for and is not to
be relied on for medical or healthcare professional advice. Please
consult your doctor or appropriate medical professional if you are
worried about your alcohol consumption in any way, and before
changing, stopping or starting a new fitness or health regime. So far
as the author is aware, the information given is correct and up to
date as at 15/03/2023. The author and publishers disclaim, as far as
the law allows, any liability arising directly or indirectly from the
use or misuse of the information contained in this book.

CONTENTS

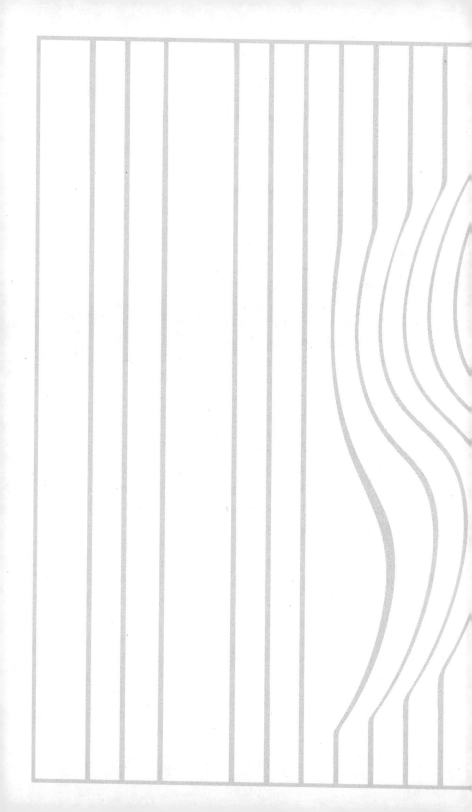

INTRODUCTION

Welcome to the World of Soberish

A NOTE FROM ME

Hello there! If you're reading this then you're interested in changing your relationship with alcohol. I'm happy to say that you've picked up the right book. My name is Kayla, and I started my own journey toward what I now call a soberish lifestyle back in 2015, when I decided that alcohol was no longer serving me in a positive way. Over the years, I'd tried many different programmes, read boat-loads of literature, threw myself into therapy (and God knows what else) trying to find the "right pathway" to heal myself. What I eventually came to learn – and what I hope to share with you through this book – is that there is no single "right way", there is only *your way*. Which is unique to you, your circumstances, your background and your future goals.

Being soberish isn't about being abstinent from alcohol, it's about writing your own narrative, finding a positive pathway to healing and taking your power back from alcohol. The world is already full of people trying to tell us what to do, who to be and how to do things; I'm not here to be one of those people. I'm simply here to share with you my experience of finding inner peace by throwing out what everyone else told me to do and choosing to do things my way – cue Frank Sinatra.

Given that we are all unique and one of a kind, it would make sense to assume that our relationship with alcohol is also unique. Working from that assumption, it wouldn't make sense to follow a strict "one-size-fits-all" programme. The soberish approach that I will be sharing in this book works like your own personal resource and toolkit buffet. You get to pick and choose what works best for you, which techniques you'd like to implement and how you'd like to move forward in changing your relationship with alcohol. I set no expectations, give you no rules to follow and only provide you with evidence-based information and real-world experiences from myself and others who have travelled their own soberish journeys. My own relationship with alcohol used to be a toxic cycle I had no idea how to break until I finally made some life-altering decisions that led me to my current lifestyle, and eventually to writing this book. That's what *Soberish* is really about: sharing my journey and guiding you on your path to creating your own.

There will be no labels, no qualifications or boxes you need to fit neatly into here. Your take on what soberish means is going to be defined by you, not by anybody else's terminology. It will be about one thing only, and that is helping you find a healthier relationship with alcohol, whatever your starting point and whether you are worried that your drinking already is a problem or just concerned that it might become one in the future.

My hope is that my science-based approach will give you permission to explore what being soberish means to you, without the pressure or expectations you may experience using other programmes. Only you know what will work for you, what motivates you and if you're truly ready to change the way you drink. My job is to give you a safe space in which to look internally and foster the confidence to forge your own path, equipped with some powerful tools that can help you do this.

On the same note, I advise that if you are alcohol dependent or drink heavily, you should seek medical assistance to map out a course of action before cutting back or stopping your use of alcohol. This will provide you with the safest experience possible. But first, I'd like to tell you a bit about my own journey, starting with how alcohol became a problem for me.

Kayla X

MY JOURNEY TO A SOBERISH LIFE

I spent the majority of my adolescent teen years feeling a bit like an outsider. I could never pinpoint exactly why I didn't feel quite like I belonged, even after I bought the "right" clothes, hung out with the seemingly "acceptable" crowd and put a whole lot of effort into getting people to like me. Picture Cady from *Mean Girls* but with blonde hair and, yes, I had literally moved from overseas too, so I was also experiencing a culture shock. I had no sense of self-identity, so I did what most 15-year-old adolescents do: I tried to fit in.

But regardless of how many friends I had, I would still walk into a party, a sleepover or a locker room and think, "No one here *really* likes me." I was extremely lonely and unsure of myself. Have you ever felt like that? The effort I was putting into being "part of" something was exhausting, and when I look back now it was almost unnatural; I was entirely out of my element, with not an ounce of authenticity in my teenage body. That was, until I found alcohol.

Now, I won't get into my very long and tumultuous relationship with alcohol, but I will tell you this. I had my first "drunk" while visiting family in Canada at age 15 and to be honest, I didn't like how it felt at all – at least to begin with. I felt out of control and confused until I realized that for the first time in my entire life I didn't feel like I wanted to crawl out of my own skin. Some people refer to this moment as "the arrival", and I'd have to agree; it finally felt as if I was at home in my own body. The normal crippling social anxiety, self-doubt and low self-esteem I felt seemed to disappear and I felt like a superhero (later supervillain) version of myself. How had I waited this long to find this feeling? *And when could I do it next?* This dangerously obsessive mindset followed me throughout my drinking career, through high school, college and eventually led me to my decision to change my relationship with alcohol for good. I was never a *let's just have one* kind of person; I was a *let's get fucked up and see what happens* kind of person. My entire high school and college experience revolved around alcohol – when could we drink, when was the next party, how could we sneak in our water bottles full of Smirnoff Raspberry into the concert or the movie theatre.

Alcohol became the glue that connected me to my social circle. That's not to say I didn't love my friends, but I often look back and wonder how much we actually had in common besides a desire to drink, party and be seen. We were all lost – I mean, who isn't at that age? – and drinking felt like a way to escape the stress, the hormones and the heartbreak. I can reflect now and see all of the places I went wrong, but then again hindsight is 20/20. I allowed my drinking and partying to take priority over my academics. Once a high-achieving, varsity athlete with scholarship opportunities, I became someone who skipped class because I was too hungover, or, worse, I'd show up drunk because I knew there was a party or a tailgate right after.

I surrounded myself with other people who drank the way I did so that I could hide in plain sight. No one from the fraternity where I was a "big sister" was going to call me out for blacking out and falling asleep in the Big Al Bar's bathroom, because they were doing the same. Without even realizing it, I found people who drank like me, which was a way to enable my drinking. Regardless of the consequences – and I promise you, there were many – nothing was going to stop me. From the time that first drink hit my lips until the day I finally started my soberish journey at age 23, alcohol was my only priority. I lost friendships, burned bridges, broke hearts, ruined relationships and, worst of all, I completely lost myself – but it didn't matter. Because when all of that regret and shame hit, the only thing I had to do was reach for a glass of wine or a bottle of gin and I knew those horrible, gut-wrenching feelings would dissipate the minute the booze hit my bloodstream.

It wasn't until a series of unfortunate, self-created events landed me into a 30-day in-patient programme in 2015 that my soberish journey really began. Even then – as I walked into rehab wearing a Victoria's Secret pink tracksuit, looking like a total asshole – I knew I wasn't ready to stop, but I did know something had to change. People who had healthy relationships with alcohol didn't end up in rehab, they didn't end up in out-patient programmes, or get underage alcohol citations. I had tried cutting back several times, and had even given it up totally for short periods, only to end up going back to my old behaviours. I just couldn't imagine a life for myself without alcohol being centre-stage.

I wish I could say that I had a great epiphany in treatment and that I left a changed young woman, but that is not my story. I will say, however, that a seed had been planted. Rehab was the first place I had the opportunity to meet other people who not only drank like me, but who recognized it was maladaptive to their lifestyle. We were all so young and damaged and just wanted to connect, and I think under different circumstances more of us would have made it out of there and stayed clean or recovered like I did. But that wasn't the case. I've lost a lot of friends to drugs and alcohol over the years, including people I spent those 30 days with.

After about a year of what I now call "sober-curiosity", spending weeks alcohol-free here and there, attending AA (Alcoholics Anonymous) meetings and going to therapy, I hit yet another rock bottom and decided it was time for me to retire completely from my drinking career. People often ask, "How did you know you were done?" and I'll be honest: I have no idea. For me, the experience was almost spiritual. Let me set the scene for you. I was driving back to Los Angeles from up north, where I lived at the time, with one of the worst hangovers of my life, trapped on the highway due to wildfires. I had no alcohol on me, so all I could do was blast my A/C and try to keep down my usual hangxiety remedy of Sprite and Powerade (which I did not). Throwing up into a large McDonalds cup in standstill traffic is a humbling experience, but then again, so is ruining your entire life for a substance that couldn't care less if you live or die. When I got back to Los Angeles, I immediately called someone I knew from rehab and went to an AA meeting, and that was the real beginning of my soberish story.

SOBERISH – A NEW APPROACH

In 2016, there was no sober/sober-curious Instagram, no online communities, no quit-lit, no sobriety- or harm-reduction-based apps – just traditional programmes like rehab and AA. I used the AA's 12-Step programme because I desperately needed community support and I wanted to change; but, if I'm being honest, I had a hard time fitting in. Now, I know every group is different, so I don't want to pigeonhole an entire movement, but I will give you my experience. At the age of 23, I had an extremely difficult time with the idea that I would never get to drink again (and I did, but more on that later). The idea of it being *forever* was extremely daunting and felt impossible. Most programmes at that time were also religiously based and I was, and still am, agnostic, so handing my power over to a "Sky Daddy" I didn't believe in was a no-go for me. The foundation of the whole programme was the 12 Steps, and if I couldn't even accept one of the first steps – about believing in a Higher Power – how was I supposed to fully commit? I hated the idea of doing anything half-assed, but I had just spent the last eight years of my life living inauthentically and I wasn't about to start this new chapter on that same note. So I only stayed for a short while.

After about two years, I decided to venture out on my own. Now, you have to understand how difficult this was, because the AA programme had been the basis for my managing to stay alcohol- and drug-free for the whole of that period, but I had hit a wall and felt stagnant in my progress. I wanted to learn more about alcohol abuse, and understand *why* I drank the way I did. I wasn't buying into the whole "you have a disease you were born with" ideology, but I was scared to leave the programme for fear of going back to old behaviours. It had been drilled into my head that if I stopped "running a programme" I would most certainly end up in "jails, institutions or death" (yes, that's a direct quote).

I eventually decided I was willing to take the chance after hearing someone at a meeting share that he didn't go to meetings anymore and how he was only there as a favour to a friend. He explained that although he didn't participate in AA anymore, it had led him to Buddhism and that is how he practised his sober journey. I was in shock after the meeting and just remember thinking to myself, "Oh my God, I can leave!"

Admittedly, in the beginning it was extremely difficult to stay on track without the structured programme I was used to, but I knew I had to carve my own path if I wanted not only to stay alcohol-free, but recover from whatever it was that had me drinking my life away in the first place. When I left the programme I was pretty much ostracized from that community. I was considered "dry" for practising abstinence with no programme, and was treated as if I was doing something wrong. I was lucky I had "normie" (people who drink) friends who supported my transition and I had found other ways of dealing with my emotions and life stressors, like becoming a fitness trainer, seeing a therapist, going back to school and beginning a yoga practice. Still, there was something missing – and that was a sense of community.

It was around 2019 when I decided to take my search for other like-minded young people to social media. It all started with a hashtag I created: #1000HoursDry. This was my attempt to challenge the people in my life and my followers to sample a sober-curious life without all the rules and restrictions traditional programming had put onto me. The idea was to set a 42-day alcohol-free challenge that was all-inclusive, which required no labelling and was focused on the benefits of not drinking, rather than a punishment- or fear-based approach.

I also figured it would be a way to meet people who already lived a no/low-alcohol lifestyle and who weren't anonymous about their experience – and I was right. Within just a few months, I had to create an entirely new Instagram page for the challenge, because so many people were interested in joining and trying it out. It was seemed surreal – *people wanting to try the alcohol-free lifestyle without being "alcoholic"*? Everything I had been taught about the binary idea of "sobriety" was thrown out the window and the idea of soberish was born. For me, being sober curious is about questioning your relationship with alcohol, while soberish invites you to begin reclaiming your power as part of that process, equipped with information and using the sorts of tools that I will be sharing in this book. (See page 78 for descriptions of some of the terms used in this book.)

Surely, I reasoned, if there were tens of thousands of people just on Instagram who were wanting to change their relationship with alcohol, there must be hundreds of thousands of people out there wanting to do the same? And the thing is, it wasn't even about sobriety in the traditional sense; it was about changing the narrative and asking yourself: "What would my life be like if I took a break from drinking or cut back?" This simple change from a fixed mindset to a growth mindset opened my eyes to an entire world of people who had been neglected and who were looking for resources and a community that didn't even exist – *yet*. I knew I needed to create a space for these individuals and that is when 1,000 Hours Dry became more than just a challenge, but a community movement dubbed "The Dry Club".

The Dry Club is a safe online space where people can explore their relationship with alcohol without judgement or fear or rejection because they don't qualify as having a "bad enough problem". Its main focus is on education, support and promoting the positive benefits of the no/low-alcohol lifestyle. Since then, I've gone on to found the Join Soberish movement – another inclusive online community dedicated to those looking to change their relationship with alcohol. Rather than fear-mongering, I want to show the fun, beneficial side of living a soberish lifestyle – and that's why this book is not about promoting abstinence as the only way or pushing the idea that you must fit into a box to question your relationship with alcohol. The point of *Soberish* is to show you that there is no one way to change your relationship with alcohol or to carve your own pathway to a healthier lifestyle. Being soberish means freeing yourself from the power alcohol holds over so many of us, forging your own path and healing in a way that works for you. To practise your journey with intention and radical honesty of self.

Before you get started on exploring the soberish techniques, it might be helpful to take a closer look at the relationship that Western society has with alcohol, to give some context.

ALCOHOL AND THE BIRTH OF DRINKING CULTURES

While alcohol has little or no place in many countries, cultures and religions around the world, it plays such a central role in some societies today that we've almost come to take its presence for granted. I don't know about you, but it seems like everywhere I go – restaurants, theatres, social gatherings, even my own living room – alcohol is there. I can't help but be painfully aware of the cascade of TV commercials, advertisements or cocktail menus displayed in front of me and I can't remember a time when it wasn't this way. Curious to know if it has always been like this, with alcohol being glamorized and used as the ultimate social lubricant, I did a little digging to find out more about our relationship with it.

Now, alcohol has literally been around forever: its documentation goes back as far as 7000 to 6600 BCE in northern China,[1] and it was used for medicinal purposes in ancient Egypt and India.[2] The Greeks and the Romans thought of it as a marker of cultural sophistication, using it socially and also in religious ceremonies, as did several Native American civilizations. Early on, however, there were warnings in most cultures against drunkenness and public displays of intoxication. But where it really seems to become more problematic is in 16th-century England, where public displays of "drunkenness" were officially deemed a crime.[3] And from there things only got worse. From the early 18th century on, the consumption of unregulated grain alcohol in Britain offered a survival mechanism of sorts to the poor and a luxury vice to the rich. In particular, the public developed a taste for gin, which had been introduced as a medicine for ailments such as indigestion and gout,[4] but which soon became increasingly popular as a cheap way to get drunk. This earned the drink the nickname "mother's ruin".

During the peak of the "Gin Craze" years, people were dying left, right and centre, with mass intoxication causing immense social problems such as violence, crime and insanity. This led the government to enact the Gin Act 1751, which was designed to reduce consumption by stopping gin distillers from selling to unlicensed merchants. It also restricted retail licenses and charged high fees to those merchants who were eligible to sell distilled spirits.[5] The Gin Act had a positive effect for a while, until the introduction of "gin palaces", which were basically luxurious gin bars. In an attempt to make gin desirable again, these bars were a way of gentrifying what had once been deemed a public concern. And it worked. Problematic drinking began to rise once more and eventually led to an upsurge of groups belonging to the Temperance Movement, which campaigned for the moderation of alcohol consumption. Since the 17th century, Temperance Movement groups had campaigned against the perils of drink. They had initially gained popularity through the Church, but some became increasingly radical over time. Many of these groups had links to political reform movements and held rallies and marches in support of "teetotalism" (complete abstinence).[6]

On the other side of the Atlantic, the Temperance Movement gained popularity in the United States during the Prohibition years of 1920 to 1933, when alcohol was banned. Even after the Prohibition era had ended, the liquor industry's fear that it might return fuelled a drive to promote drinking in a new way. Those fears were not unjustified, because during the late 1930s two fifths of Americans surveyed still supported national Prohibition.[7] So now, rather than focusing their promotion efforts on the rough saloon culture of the time, brewers and distillers targeted a larger new audience with propaganda, creating a "cocktail culture" of glamour, wealth and sophistication around alcohol, which caught on in Britain too. There were catchy slogans such as "Guinness is good for you" and colourful adverts showing smiling, well-groomed men and women. Suddenly, booze was being pushed by sellers in both the United States and Britain as the ultimate social lubricant. And people bought into it, hook, line and sinker.

You may be thinking, "Well, that was like one hundred years ago, things are obviously different now!" But the truth is that not much has changed. If anything, things have only gotten worse. Today, consumers are being flooded with alcohol advertising in all forms of media, including ones that didn't exist until relatively recently, such as the internet and social media platforms. Besides this, most of us were never properly educated on the negative effects of alcohol, because the information isn't readily available or taught. Worst of all, there's usually very little information about the risks or side-effects on the labelling of the products themselves.

Alcohol is manufactured and sold without a required nutrition label or sufficiently detailed health-warning label. No FDA or FSA regulation is required in the US or the UK. In the US, the current mandatory government warning reads: "(1) According to the Surgeon General, women should not drink alcoholic beverages during pregnancy because of the risk of birth defects. (2) Consumption of alcoholic beverages impairs your ability to drive a car or operate machinery, and may cause health problems."[8] Outdated is an understatement. Since the introduction of the Surgeon General's warning in the mid-1980s, we know for certain that drinking while pregnant can cause birth defects such as foetal alcohol syndrome and that alcohol is directly correlated with a smorgasbord of health problems such as heart disease, liver disease, mental health issues, addiction and seven different types of cancer.[9] In the UK, the labelling policy is even less informative, reading: "Please Drink Responsibly. UK Chief Medical Officers recommend men do not regularly exceed 3–4 units daily and women, 2–3 units daily. Avoid alcohol if pregnant or trying to conceive."[10]

I say this not to scare you but to open your eyes. I'm a firm believer that, as adults, we have the right to do whatever we want with our bodies and we have the right to consume whatever we want. Where there is a problem is the lack of available knowledge and the clear misrepresentation of alcohol in advertising and the media. As consumers we deserve the right to *informed consent*, meaning that we should be given sufficient information on the potential risks of what we are putting into our bodies. If there is no updated warning label on alcohol, the way there is on tobacco products, no nutrition label as required by regulated government agencies, and advertisers can continue to promote only the glamorous side of alcohol, how are we expected to know the potential health risks to drinking? Well, it's a trick question, because we aren't.

THE BIRTH OF A BINARY SOBRIETY

The Prohibition era was extremely hard on habitual drinkers, but not because they were cut off from alcohol. You and I know that if we want a drink bad enough, we'll find it, and they did too. The real problem was that the individuals who recognized their drinking was destructive were limited in terms of their treatment resources. The programmes that were available, such as the Washington Total Abstinence Movement, asked for complete sobriety, which was a deterrent for many. On top of this, during the US Prohibition, the inebriate asylums (institutes specifically designed to treat alcoholism) had closed and other self-help societies had withered away.[11] That is, until 1935, when these conditions gave birth to the self-help group we now know as Alcoholics Anonymous (AA).[12] Their approach to alcoholism was more radical than that of many societies and deeply influenced by the Washington Total Abstinence Movement, which in turn had originally sprung from the Temperance Movement. AA membership rapidly rose, with groups spreading across the States, and in November 1948 the first AA meeting took place in Manchester, England.

AA and rehabilitation facilities drew a rigid line between those who could moderate their drinking and "compulsive drinkers" who could not, in this way creating a societal cognitive distortion of black-and-white thinking when it came to alcohol misuse, or alcohol use disorder (AUD) – the term now used to describe a problematic pattern of alcohol use. Although the concept's principal aim was to encourage sympathy for "alcoholics", its result was ironically to open the door to drinking by everyone else.[13] The resultant binary way of thinking created the belief that you have to be alcohol dependent "to have a real problem", or to be a compulsive drinker in order to seek help or even question your relationship with alcohol, when this couldn't be farther from the truth.

Today, more and more of us are revaluating the role of alcohol in our lives. In fact, the evidence suggests that alcohol consumption is falling among the younger generations in both Britain and the United States, and that we are no longer buying into all of the myths that are propagated around it.[14,15] Contrary to what most of us have been shown through mainstream media, like many other maladaptive disorders the misuse of alcohol can be placed on a wide spectrum. This challenges the depiction of drinking in movies such as *Country Strong*, *A Star is Born* or *The Girl on the Train*, for example, which portray the drinker as a full-blown "alcoholic", playing deeper into the narrative that alcohol misuse is a black-and-white issue. And that narrative is only perpetuated by the limited options available for those of us who are struggling – like detox, in-patient treatment, out-patient programmes and 12-Step peer-support groups – which all promote abstinence as the only pathway.

But there are alternative ways to address alcohol use. The current *Diagnostic and Statistical Manual of Mental Disorders* (DSM-5) takes a slightly different approach. The DSM-5 is the handbook used by healthcare professionals in the United States and much of the world as the authoritative guide to the diagnosis of mental disorders, and it states that individuals can have a problem with alcohol that ranges from mild to moderate to severe. Knowing this can help you to open your mind to the idea that having a problem with alcohol doesn't have to look like the stereotypical homeless man under the bridge, or the housewife who can always be found with a martini in hand. Most of us struggling or questioning our relationship with alcohol appear perfectly fine from the outside: our lives are functioning, we have careers we enjoy and we've never experienced anyone telling us we need to drink less. When it comes to your own relationship with alcohol, realize that you may be asking yourself the wrong questions here. The questions shouldn't be, "Am I an alcoholic?" or "Do I have alcohol use disorder?" The questions you should be asking yourself are these:

* ★ "Is alcohol serving my life in a positive way?"
* ★ "Is it helping or hindering my goals?"
* ★ "What would my ideal life look like – and what place does alcohol have in that life?"

In the chapters that follow, I am going to support you in finding your own answers.

SETTING THE INTENTION BEHIND YOUR SOBERISH JOURNEY

With anything we do – drinking, eating, exercising – we should always be thinking of the intention behind our actions. Many of us tend to get so caught up in doing things aimlessly, or because we've always done it that way before, that we forget *why* we are doing it in the first place. So before we go any further, let's put some thought into why you are reading this book, and what you hope to gain from it along the way. In short, let's set your intention for reading *Soberish* and write this down.

When setting an intention, you want to create a successful roadmap that will bring you to the outcome you desire. The fact is that when you set specific intentions, you are more likely to achieve them. I personally use the EEE model of goal- and intention-setting, because it's all about turning our intentions into successful outcomes. This model stands for the following:

★ **Enlightening:** Ideally, our intentions should enlighten us with respect to our ultimate goal and help us gain a deeper insight into our strengths and weaknesses. By setting specific intentions, we can prioritize these according to our needs at the time. Perhaps you're reading this book, for example, because you'd like to have a healthier relationship with alcohol and ultimately perform better in your career. Both are great intentions, but putting them down on paper will show you a hierarchy you may not have seen before: that you must prioritize changing your relationship with alcohol first in order to increase your career performance.

★ **Encouraging:** We all need motivation – I certainly do. Especially when it comes to doing difficult things like changing your relationship with alcohol. When we have set intentions we can feel more confident about having a game plan and not going into what we are doing blind. Research has shown that we are 76 per cent more likely to achieve our goals if we write them down.[16] (We look at goal-setting in more detail in chapter 4.)

★ **Enabling:** Setting an intention for what you hope to get out of reading this book will enable you to strengthen your intention- and goal-setting skills, which will come in handy for chapter 15, "Beating Backsliding Behaviours", when we will be looking again at the long-term goals we hope to achieve through this new lifestyle.

SET YOUR INTENTIONS

Based on the EEE method, let's set some clear intentions for why you are reading this book and what you hope to gain from it. Please tick any intentions that apply to you:

- ☐ To gain understanding of how alcohol impacts my body and brain.
- ☐ To learn how to cut back my drinking.
- ☐ To find answers to why I drink the way I do.
- ☐ To learn healthier coping skills for dealing with uncomfortable emotions.
- ☐ To improve my relationships.
- ☐ To build a foundation to a soberish life.
- ☐ To become a better version of myself.
- ☐ To have guidance on the direction I should take my drinking.
- ☐ To have more resources for adopting a soberish lifestyle.

Now, write down any intentions of your own that come to mind.

★ ....

★ ....

★ ....

★ ....

Keep referring back to these intentions as you progress through this book and particularly when drawing up your soberish Plan of Action in chapter 4 and creating your toolkit in Part Two.

• •

GETTING STARTED

It's time to get started on finding out what soberish could mean for you and what that might look like in your everyday life. All of the findings and tools that I will be sharing with you are based on the latest scientific research and the experience of experts. (If you want to discover more, please turn to listings in the Endnotes and the Resources sections at the back of this book.)

In Part One, we're going to be doing some groundwork by considering the physical effects of booze, the impact of these on the brain and our thinking, and how this in turn may affect our relationship with alcohol. Then there are exercises designed to help you find out what kind of drinker you are (you might be surprised) and to start taking back control of your narrative by setting some goals and creating your own Plan of Action. As some of these practices involve writing stuff down, you may find it useful to have a special journal or notebook to use alongside your soberish journey. You'll also find insights shared by members of my soberish grapevine who have been along this path before you, and – like me – are there to support you.

In Part Two, it's time to assemble your soberish toolkit. I'm going to introduce you to a whole heap of fun and useful practices, from diet to manifesting, mindfulness to the cold exposure method, and many more. These are designed to help you connect with your mind and body in supportive ways, and are based on techniques that have been scientifically proven to be beneficial.

Part Three is about putting those tools to work, learning to spot backsliding behaviours, practising self-care and nurturing your own happiness. It's about taking back the power from alcohol and channelling that energy into creating the future you want. This is where the adventure really starts.

Now, my approach may be nuanced or frowned upon by other programmes, but I'm not here to serve those people: I am here to serve you and your soberish journey. Perhaps you are experimenting with sober-curiosity, cutting back or trying a dry challenge to see how you like it — I don't care! As long as you are healing and the intention behind what you are doing is allowing yourself to evolve and grow, I believe in my heart of hearts that you are on the path the universe has set out for you.

Let's get started!

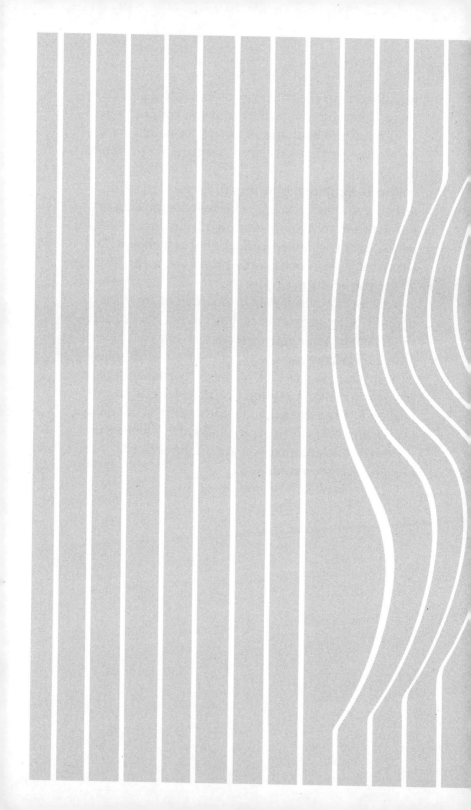

Soberish – A New Approach

SOBERISH – A NEW APPROACH

In the beginning, changing your relationship with alcohol can feel a lot like you're giving up a huge part of your life. No matter your reason, the change in lifestyle and the stigmatization put on you by society can have you questioning your decision, but I've yet to come across anyone who has regretted following this path. Rather than focusing on what you might be missing out on, it's important we shift gears to look at the benefits of drinking less.

To start to do this, I would like to introduce you to a key player in your life: your wonderful brain. You likely already know how alcohol can affect your thinking – from obsessing about when it's cocktail hour or booze o'clock, to coping with the effects of a hangover. That's why we're going to start by taking a closer look at the effects of booze on the brain, and also how the nature of the brain itself can help shape the future course of our relationship with alcohol.

Once we've familiarized ourselves with some of the ways in which alcohol can affect our thinking, we're going to look at how the language used around drinking can impact us in unhelpful ways too – and how to reclaim our narrative.

Next, based on the principle that knowledge is power, I'll be inviting you to consider your own drinking patterns. Self-awareness is key on this journey, so we'll get to work on finding out what motivates you and setting some goals for you to work toward. You'll also be creating your own Plan of Action. As you're about to discover, Part One is all about doing the groundwork.

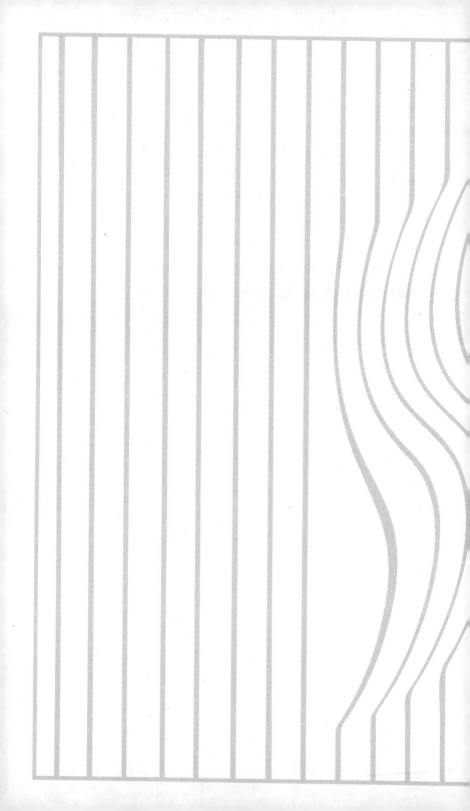

CHAPTER 1

Understanding the Brain–Booze Connection

Until the late 20th century, it was widely believed
that our brains could change only during adolescence.
This implied that the brain didn't have the ability to
grow and reorganize its neural networks after a certain
age, which meant we were stuck with what we had.
Thankfully, research on neuroplasticity in adults proved
this old theory wrong. If you're unfamiliar with the
term "neuroplasticity", it basically means the brain's
ability to adapt and change based on your current
experiences. This term is very important to this book,
because of the role neuroplasticity plays in both the
causation of alcohol misuse and the ability to change
the way we consume.

When we drink, alcohol creates or strengthens neural
pathways in the brain that trigger our reward system
neurotransmitters, such as dopamine. This is why the
first drink usually feels quite relaxing or pleasurable.
Over time, the more we consume the stronger these
pathways become, making it more difficult for our brains
to imagine virtually anything else as being as pleasurable
or stress-reducing. Think of these neural pathways acting
like hiking trails in the forest. The more often you take
a specific trail, the more likely you are to continue to
use it, because it's *familiar*. Each time you hike this trail
your muscle memory becomes stronger and even more
automatic – you know where the trees hang low and
where to avoid small creeks, so it's easier to navigate.
As you continue to take this trail, it grows larger from
each use, until eventually you don't even bother with
new trails because this one seems to get the job done.
In fact, you may even have tried to use new trails, only
to find they were too difficult or provoked anxiety
because you hadn't taken them before – so you turn
back to use your old, seemingly reliable trail.

This is what happens to your neural pathways when
you drink. No matter your reason, whether it's about

reducing stress, loneliness or socializing with friends, you continue to strengthen the neural pathways that cue you to drink, which in turn atrophies your other, healthier pathways. "One version of neuroplasticity is developing a tolerance, where your brain has adapted and you now need more alcohol to achieve the same result. For example, you need more wine to feel relaxed at night," explains Gillian Tietz, former biochemist and host of popular podcast *Sober Powered*, when I speak with her over Zoom.[1]

Like the hiking trails, your brain begins to rely on your drinking pathways solely to give you that dopamine boost, making it seemingly impossible to choose a different activity when you're feeling the urge to drink. So if you've been trying to cut back or quit for a while now, but keep falling back into old habits, it's because these extremely strong neural pathways are overpowering your weaker ones. This isn't a question of willpower or your desire to change, because if you're reading this book then we both know you want this. What it is about is swimming against the tide and using neuroplasticity in your favour. So how can you accelerate the process of creating and strengthening new neural pathways that don't involve drinking? Well, we can stop reinforcing our drinking pathways and we begin taking our new ones to the gym by using healthier coping mechanisms. (With this in mind, we will be building our own toolkit in Part Two, so stay tuned.)

LEVELS OF RISK AND ALCOHOL

Outside of changing your neural pathways in harmful ways and potentially leading you to develop alcohol use disorder, alcohol can have extremely harmful effects on the brain if consumed at high levels over a long period of time or through binge-drinking. To gain a little more insight into the sort of quantities that are thought to be relatively low risk, check out the chart below:

Country	Women	Men
USA	<7 drinks per week	<14 drinks per week
UK	<14 drinks per week	<14 drinks per week
Australia	<10 drinks per week	<10 drinks per week
Canada	<10 drinks per week	<15 drinks per week
France	<10 drinks per week	<10 drinks per week
Germany	<5 drinks per week	<10 drinks per week
Spain	<7 drinks per week	<14 drinks per week

Figure 1. low-risk drinking quantities in select Westernized countries.

You may wonder why there is a discrepancy in the numbers. The answer is that each country has based their current guidelines on their own evidence-based trials.[2] Reasons for the differences could be dependent on the drinking culture, the drink size and strength or methods of measuring alcohol, among other reasons.[3]

WHY THE FIGURES DIFFER BETWEEN MEN AND WOMEN

Gender is a very nuanced subject, so for our purposes it's worth clarifying that the figures for low-risk and high-risk drinking simply relate to the biological sex of the body a person was born with. According to the CDC and National Institute of Alcoholism and Alcohol Use Disorder (NIAAA) in the United States, there is significant scientific evidence to back up the claim that men and women should consume alcohol at different levels. There are four major reasons, including:

① **Water content:** On average, a female body contains a lower percentage of water than a male one, meaning women can get intoxicated faster. Because there is less water to dilute the alcohol in a woman's body, the result is a higher alcohol concentration in the blood.[4] This is due to females having a higher percentage of body fat. Body size and shape and the balance of muscle and fat can all affect the percentage of water in a person's body.[5]

② **Chemical composition:** Compared to men, women have lower levels of alcohol dehydrogenase (ADH), a chemical found in the liver that aids the body in breaking down and metabolizing toxins such as alcohol. Because of this, women tend to absorb more alcohol into their bloodstream, and it tends to remain there longer.[6]

③ **Weight:** Metabolizing alcohol is directly connected to how much we weigh. In general, women tend to weigh less than men and have less tissue in their bodies to absorb alcohol. Because women also have less ADH in their stomach than men, they are less able to metabolize alcohol. So even if a man and woman with the same body weight were to ingest the same amount of alcohol, the woman will have a higher Blood Alcohol Content (BAC) than the man.

④ **Hormones:** Hormonal differences may also play a role in how alcohol affects the body.[7] Some studies suggest that blood-alcohol concentrations in women are at their highest directly before the menstrual cycle begins and at their lowest on the first day after.

Of course, this isn't even going into all the other physical effects that alcohol misuse can have on both men and women, such as different types of cancer (including breast, mouth, head and neck, liver and bowel cancers), and conditions ranging from stroke, infertility, depression and dementia.[8] Other types of risk include injury, potential violence, unsafe sex, the loss of belongings and having to take unplanned time off work or study.[9] While some health conditions may take a while to develop before they are detected, whatever your gender, the effects of alcohol on the brain can often be felt relatively quickly, in a variety of different ways.

THE DANGER ZONE

Unlike other substances and chemicals, alcohol can penetrate our blood-brain barrier (BBB), an immunological feature of the human central nervous system. Composed of many cell types, the BBB's job is to defend our brain against any disease-causing pathogens and toxins that may be present in our blood.[10] However, alcohol is still able to cross through the BBB via our blood circulation into our brain cells.[11] This can lead to the death of brain cells, which can cause brain damage. "Alcohol is dehydrating and shrinks the brain by causing neurons and the connections between neurons to lose water. This can impact the way the brain functions," Gillian Tietz explains to me.[12] Alcohol also causes reduction in white and grey matter (white matter is a large network in the brain that allows communication between different areas of grey matter, where information is processed).[13] Damage to the brain can therefore lead to the following:

★ **Lack of self-awareness:** You may fail to identify your emotions and how they impact your daily actions or those around you. You find it difficult to identify your patterns of behaviours and thinking. You may tend to experience more negative emotions than positive.

★ **Impulsivity:** You lack control over your decision-making and tend to act without thinking. You may be easily distracted or quick to anger or to feel overcome by your emotions generally.

★ **Lack of clarity:** You may not have a clear life plan because you are constantly making changes in your life. These changes can cause you stress and anxiety. You tend to question yourself, a lot.

★ **Less ability to regulate emotions:** Referred to as dysregulation, you may lack the ability to manage your emotional responses or reactions in an appropriate manner. Less ability to regulate your emotions also means larger and more frequent mood swings.

★ **Memory loss:** Excessive drinking can destroy the brain tissue and disrupt the ability to form new long-term memories. You may also experience "blackouts" or "brownouts" where parts or all of the memory from the night before are gone.

A SEVEN-DAY MINI CHALLENGE

Consider whether you have recently or ever noticed any of the symptoms listed above. You may have experienced them without even knowing their source. To find out more, let's try a mini challenge to see if there could be a correlation between the symptoms and your drinking habits.

I'd like you to go alcohol-free for seven days straight. Before you begin, note down the most common symptoms in your day-to-day life when drinking.

Write down at the end of each evening whether you experience any of the listed symptoms, or observe any improvements in them.

At the end of the seventh day, evaluate how you feel. Did any of the symptoms listed begin to dissipate after you stopped drinking? What other improvements did you notice?

If you don't make it through the whole seven days without drinking, please don't beat yourself up about it. We're only at the very start of your soberish journey, so there will be plenty more opportunities to have another go at this mini challenge.

ANHEDONIA VERSUS THE PINK CLOUD

Now, in the beginning of your soberish journey you may experience one of these two very different states: either anhedonia or what's known as "the pink cloud".

Let's start with the second one, if only because it sounds nicer.

The "pink cloud" is an old-school term for the euphoric feeling some people get in early sobriety. While there's no way to know if you'll be someone who experiences this, I was lucky in that I did. However, there are a combination of factors that may lead to a higher chance of catching your own pink cloud.

The first factor is medication. If you are someone who currently takes antidepressants such as selective serotonin reuptake inhibitors (SSRIs) and serotonin-norepinephrine reuptake inhibitor drugs (SNRIs) or an antipsychotic for a mental health disorder, you may be more likely to experience the pink cloud. This is because when you stop or significantly reduce your drinking, your medication is actually able to do its job. To put it simply, when you drink on your medication, you reduce its effectiveness. On top of this, mixing meds with alcohol can also worsen your disorder symptoms and cause potential dangerous interactions.[14]

I was someone who had direct experience with this, as I used benzodiazepines for my panic attacks and took a SNRI for my obsessive compulsive disorder (more on which later) for almost five years while still consuming alcohol. I had blackouts almost every time I drank because I was mixing two highly dangerous substances. And it also led to other high-risk situations such as drinking and driving, sleeping with strangers and alcohol poisoning. The irony of it all was that I was drinking and misusing my anti-anxiety medication to avoid my panic attacks when, in reality, it was my using alcohol that was causing them to happen so frequently. Once I decided to stop drinking for a period to rewire my system, it was as if I was experiencing life with fresh eyes, when really I was just finally allowing my medication to do its job.

Another factor that may lead to the pink cloud is your healing process. How much work you put into this journey directly correlates to exactly what you will get out of it, so the harder you try to create those new neural pathways, the more likely you are to feel the benefits of being soberish more quickly. Using your soberish toolkit, finding a strong support system, and creating a self-care routine are all examples of ways you can put yourself in a better position to see your new lifestyle from an optimistic standpoint.

On the other side of the pendulum is anhedonia, which refers to the reduced ability to experience pleasure due to chemical imbalance caused by alcohol misuse.[15] We may experience anhedonia when our pleasure baseline is out of whack. Similar to those neuro hiking trails that I mentioned earlier, our pleasure baseline is directly impacted by alcohol misuse and is reinforced negatively each time we choose to drink.

To illustrate this, I want you to imagine a plate covered like tapas in mini versions of all the things that bring you joy and pleasure. We can use mine for visualization purposes. Here I am, holding a plate full of representations of my most beloved hobbies and relationships – my girl gang, yoga, my exercise boot camp, meditation, walking my dog, nonfiction books on psychology and alcohol. Now, before I adopted a negative relationship with drinking, all of these things brought me happiness, stress-relief and peace. But over time, as I began to drink more and turned to alcohol in unhealthy ways, my baseline began to change and my plate began to shrink. It started off slow: I began to prioritize drinking and going out with friends more, so naturally the other activities fell off the plate.

The longer I drank and the more booze I consumed, the smaller my plate got until there was only room for one thing – alcohol. I had prioritized drinking over everything else. I'd used alcohol to have fun, to destress and to self-medicate so often that I'd completely atrophied my other hobbies' neural pathways. My brain had forgotten that alcohol wasn't the only thing that could bring me joy.

In order for me to create a bigger plate and rebalance my pleasure baseline, I had to start focusing on recreating those old pathways and allowing alcohol's pathway to dissipate. I had to show up to yoga class and commit to a new meditation practice even when it wasn't making me feel any better at first, because as my plate began to grow over time, so did my ability to feel happiness and relief from other activities. I had to remember this was a marathon, not a sprint. This is obviously easier said than done, which is why we will be creating a toolkit together in Part Two of this book, where I will be introducing you to a range of supportive activities that you can add to your own plate.

DO NOT MIX: ALCOHOL AND MENTAL HEALTH

Similar to the differences in how men and women metabolize alcohol, those who suffer from a mental health disorder are at greater risk of misusing alcohol.[16] Both your mental health and your likelihood of developing alcohol use disorder are based on a combination of your genetics and your environment. According to Gillian Tietz, "Everyone starts out with a specific baseline of neurons, neurotransmitters, endorphins and hormones. We are all different."[17] All-important neurotransmitters are chemicals that play a major role in regulating necessary functions in our body such as our mood, digestion, sleep and early human development.[18] Everyone has a different starting baseline depending on their chemical makeup and this is what can put some of us at a higher chance of developing a problematic relationship with alcohol.

I'll give you a personal example. I mentioned briefly that I suffer from obsessive compulsive disorder (OCD), a common and very debilitating anxiety disorder. Recent studies suggest that one of the causes of OCD may be due to the dysregulation of the neurotransmitter glutamate.[19] Research has shown that those with OCD seem to have higher levels of glutamate,[20] which may be the cause of some of the symptoms of the disorder such as compulsions, anxiety and panic attacks. All of this is to say that I started off life with a lower baseline because of my natural internal chemical imbalance.

The more dysregulation we start with, the more imbalance we have to work against when using coping mechanisms, medication, proper nutrition and other tools, such as those we're going to be looking at in Part Two. Alcohol further disrupts the chemical balance in our bodies, which can cause problems for those without mental health disorders and even worse symptoms for those who do. Opposite is a line graph to illustrate this.

As you can see, we all start with a baseline that represents our most balanced self. (As mentioned, some baselines are lower than others, but let's just use this general baseline for now to keep things simple.) Over time, your baseline will begin to decrease with the continued misuse of alcohol. This is because the systems in your body are becoming dysregulated. When we drink, we see an increase in our baseline for a short period because of the release of dopamine activated by

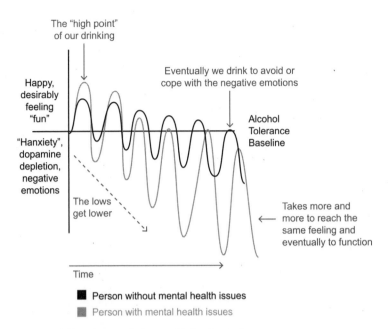

Figure 2. The chemicals in our body throughout our alcohol journey.

alcohol. But what goes up must come down and after the short-lived positive effects of alcohol have worn off, we are left at an even lower point than our initial baseline because of dopamine depletion.[21]

Alcohol is categorized as a depressant drug, which is why it causes your pleasure neurotransmitter, dopamine, to decrease after use. This is why you may feel sad, moody, sleepy or experience hangxiety – a term coined to express the anxiety sometimes experienced after drinking alcohol. This entire process is magnified for those who already suffer from a mental health disorder and are starting with a lower baseline. As time goes on and you continue to drink, your system becomes more and more imbalanced, causing your original baseline to lower. This is why you find you need to consume higher levels of alcohol more often to experience the same effects; this is your tolerance increasing.

As you can see on the graph, the longer and more you continue to drink, the further your baseline drops, making it even harder to reach a point at which you find pleasure from drinking. Eventually, you need to drink just to reach your initial baseline, which is where alcohol dependence steps into play. "The lower your baseline continues to drop, the more likely you are to experience alcohol-induced depression, anxiety or even psychosis," explains Gillian Tietz, "and you don't need to suffer from any mental health condition to experience these temporary effects."[22]

The good news is that for those of us who suffer from alcohol-induced depression, anxiety or psychosis, drinking less or quitting can alleviate the issue.[23] For those suffering from a mental health disorder like myself, changing your relationship with alcohol can help you manage your symptoms much more easily and allow your medication to work with full force. My overall consensus would be that if you're looking to improve your mental health, it may be a good time to consider drinking less and adopting a soberish lifestyle.

THE DIATHESIS–STRESS MODEL

Until fairly recently, what is now clinically referred to as alcohol use disorder was called "alcoholism". Now, I'm sure you're familiar with the term and its negative connotations – like the image of a homeless individual under a bridge or that distant cousin who can't seem to get their life together. The term carries a lot of weight and is linked to the binary idea that we somehow need to "qualify" to be an alcoholic. While this is problematic for a number of reasons, one of the most significant is the worldwide view that having a problem with alcohol is a disease, something we're born with and doomed to have, no matter what. I'm calling bullshit. While severe alcohol use over time can *cause* disease of the brain, leading to conditions such as Wernicke-Korsakoff syndrome, nobody is born with a hereditary gene marker labelled "alcoholic". As explained to me by former biochemist Gillian Tietz, alcohol use disorder is caused by both genetic and environmental factors.

Alcohol use disorder and other substance use disorders can be best explained, in my opinion, by the diathesis–stress model of addiction. This theory states that these disorders are "a combination of heredity (genetic), environment (epigenetic) and pharmacologic factors that result in the hijacking of the survival mechanism of the brain."[24] In other words, you can develop a problem with alcohol because of a large combination of different genetic predisposing factors and environmental stressors that happen over time. For an illustration of this, see the following drawing:

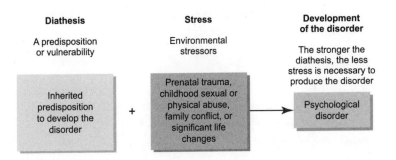

Diathesis	Stress	Development of the disorder
A predisposition or vulnerability	Environmental stressors	The stronger the diathesis, the less stress is necessary to produce the disorder
Inherited predisposition to develop the disorder	+ Prenatal trauma, childhood sexual or physical abuse, family conflict, or significant life changes	→ Psychological disorder

Figure 3. The diathesis–stress model.

It seems that alcohol use disorder is a case of both nature and nurture, in which genetic factors and other considerations can potentially create a diathesis, or predisposition, toward it if the circumstances are right.

PREDISPOSITIONS OR VULNERABILITIES

Let's take a closer look at some of the ingredients that may give a person an inherited predisposition to develop alcohol use disorder – the diathesis or "nature" part of the model.

Baselines of neurochemicals

We've already touched on one significant factor – how every person starts with a unique baseline of neurochemicals such as GABA (the primary inhibitory neurotransmitter in the brain), glutamate (the most abundant neurotransmitter in the brain) and serotonin (the feel-good hormone that carries messages between nerve cells). Depending on your starting baseline you may be at higher risk of developing a problematic relationship with alcohol. For example, if you are like me and suffer from a genetic mental health disorder where your natural levels of specific neurotransmitters are lower than average, you may have an inherited disposition to alcohol use disorder.

Tolerance

Alcohol tolerance develops over a period of time when an individual drinks frequently. Your tolerance is changed in a negative capacity when you need to drink more to feel the same effects; for example, it takes you three beers to feel "buzzed" when it used to only take one. This can create a vulnerability toward the general overconsumption of alcohol. Moreover, research has found that the enzyme cytochrome

(CYP2E1) plays a role in ethanol sensitivity in the brain.[25] As author and biomedical researcher Dr Samir Zakhari notes, higher levels of CYP2E1 contribute to a higher tolerance, therefore promoting more alcohol consumption in the individual.[26]

Genetic alcohol metabolism

There are two specific genes that research has found directly affect your risk of AUD: alcohol dehydrogenase (ADH1B) and aldehyde dehydrogenase (ALDH2).[27] These genes impact how the body metabolizes and processes alcohol. Different variations of these genes can cause a build-up of acetaldehyde, an organic chemical that results from alcohol being metabolized in the body. If you have certain mutations of ADH1B and ALDH2, you may be prone to having higher levels of acetaldehyde in your system after drinking. Higher levels of acetaldehyde can cause facial flushing, rapid heart rate and nausea.[28] People with these mutations tend to be at lower risk because of their bodies' natural aversion to alcohol. As we discussed on page 9, women in particular have lower levels of (ADH) and because of this, tend to absorb more alcohol into their bloodstream, and it tends to remain there longer.[29]

Flexible thinking

Cognitive flexibility is your ability to adapt your behaviour based on changes to your environment. Some people are born with more flexibility than others, and the less flexible you are in your thinking, the harder it is for you to adapt your behaviour (your drinking) to what you're experiencing (i.e. the consequences). Chronic heavy drinking changes our behavioural control system in the brain from being flexible and goal-directed to habitual and inflexible. Despite the same negatives showing up over and over, this inflexibility prevents us from recognizing the cause and effect of our drinking. Instead, we carry on drinking, believing this time will surely be different.

Personality

Certain personality traits can also be a factor in your predisposition to AUD. Findings published by the International Institute of Anticancer Research explain how these traits can include impulsivity, disinhibition and neuroticism.[30] A sign of impulsivity in an individual can be an inability to regulate their behaviours or emotions. When someone has issues with impulsivity, they are more likely to participate in risky behaviours such as excessive alcohol use.[31] Similarly, disinhibition can result from poor risk assessment and an inability to show self-restraint. High levels of neuroticism, including anger, anxiety, self-consciousness, irritability, emotional instability and depression, all put you at a higher risk of developing problematic drinking.

Potential environmental factors

Now we turn to the "nurture" part of the diathesis–stress model – the factors in our circumstances that could combine with our genetics and personality traits to make it more likely that we will develop AUD, for example. However, it doesn't necessarily mean we will. As I said, I absolutely don't believe anyone is doomed to become an "alcoholic". All the same, it's worth becoming self-aware and thinking about any aspects in your circumstances that could trigger a predisposition to developing the disorder. That's why, instead of listing a load of scientific facts, this time I'm going to ask you to have a think about your own situation too:

★ **Childhood experiences:** How were you brought up? Did your parents drink? What sort of attitude did the adults around you have to alcohol? What did you observe? How old were you when you had your first drink and what was it like? In what ways could this affect how you feel about drinking now?

★ **Coping mechanisms:** What sort of strategies were you taught to help you deal with difficult situations? For example, were you taught it was OK to ask for help? If something went wrong or became upsetting for you, how did you deal with that – by trying to fix things, changing your outlook on the situation or by looking for a distraction from it?

★ **Trauma:** Trauma is an emotional response to distressing situations. These can range from one-off events such as a crime, an accident or a natural disaster, to causes of ongoing stress such as abuse or emotional upheaval. Trauma may disrupt your body's natural balance.[32] Recent research described by award-winning health writer Karina Margit Erdelyi suggests that trauma can even impact people at an epigenetic level and be passed down through families in the ways their genes are expressed.[33] Have you experienced trauma in any way? How have you dealt with this?

★ **Chronic stress:** Have you ever experienced continuous stress? This might have been through your work if you have a particularly demanding job like, say, a lawyer or doctor. Or perhaps you just feel deeply dissatisfied or unhappy in a relationship. Chronic stress can be exhausting and leave us feeling stuck and unable to change.[34] Increased alcohol use can be a symptom of this condition.

★ **Socioeconomic status:** What resources do you have access to? Socioeconomic status refers to your education, income and type of job, which may affect the sort of opportunities that are likely to be available to you. Do you feel in control of your own choices, or that opportunities are heavily curtailed for you in some way because of who you are?

BREAKING THE CYCLE

Changing our relationship with alcohol can bring up a lot of anticipatory anxiety about the future. Sometimes we stay in the same unhealthy cycle simply because it's become a habit that is comfortable to us in a strange way. Almost like a trauma bond with alcohol – an unhealthy connection between an abused person and their abuser. However, it can bring a sense of ease and empowerment when we begin to understand that there are many mechanisms at work internally in our body systems that are perpetuating this cycle, and that it isn't about a lack of willpower. Becoming aware of the cycle is the first step to practising acceptance and leaning into change.

I'm sure most of us have experienced the exact same cycle I'm talking about. We take a drink, enjoy ourselves for a bit and then – BAM! – we go over our limit, we start to get emotional or put ourselves into high-risk situations. Once the alcohol has worn off, we are left with a hangover, feelings of shame or embarrassment and the occasional apology tour because we can't quite remember what we did the night before. We feel gross emotionally and physically and we vow to never drink again, or at least to take a break. Then, by the end of the day (or sometimes days), we begin to feel better and that little voice in our head starts to say, "Well, was it really that bad?" And we start the cycle over. Sound familiar?

You're probably wondering why you can't seem to break the habit no matter how many times you promise yourself or your loved ones that it won't happen again. And while there is no one answer, this type of inflexible thinking and behaviour can once again be linked back to alcohol's impact on the brain.

One of the characteristics of alcohol misuse is impaired thinking. This impairment can cause cognitive inflexibility, reflecting our inability to update the information that guides our decision-making.[35] To illustrate this, imagine your brain acts like the hard drive of a computer: when you consume high levels

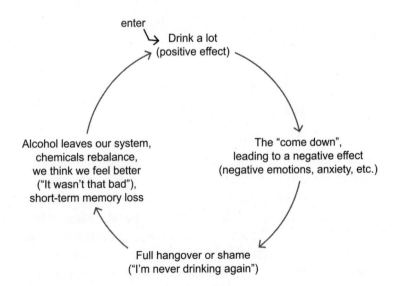

enter
Drink a lot
(positive effect)

Alcohol leaves our system,
chemicals rebalance,
we think we feel better
("It wasn't that bad"),
short-term memory loss

The "come down",
leading to a negative effect
(negative emotions, anxiety, etc.)

Full hangover or shame
("I'm never drinking again")

Figure 4. The drinking cycle.

of alcohol you begin to damage that hard drive. Now, instead of storing accurate information as it's being processed in real time, your hard drive begins to malfunction, causing your brain to be unable to update things such as your negative memories from drinking – "I wasn't that bad, was I?" (Cue side eye.)

I was very guilty of this sort of impaired thinking when I was drinking. I was also extremely impulsive, another characteristic of alcohol misuse. This impulsivity led me to make decisions I normally wouldn't have made if I'd been sober, and to act before thinking, which kept me in an unhealthy cycle. Even when I was in my sober-curious phase, I found it really difficult to wrap my head around the idea of not drinking anymore, or at least drinking significantly less. My whole lifestyle was intertwined with alcohol. It wasn't until I switched my perspective to what I could gain from ditching booze, instead of what I was losing or missing out on, that I was able to go from contemplation to action mode.

THE LIMITLESS BENEFITS OF BEING SOBERISH

By now you have a better idea of the ways in which alcohol can impact your brain, body and mental health. And while some of these facts can seem daunting, the good news is that, thanks to neuroplasticity, you can reverse the damage with a few behavioural changes. In the same way the brain can create neural pathways that cue us to drink, you can reverse these and create new neural pathways that will lead you to healthier coping mechanisms. All you need is patience, practice and, of course, your soberish toolkit, which we'll be looking at in Part Two. Here are some reasons why being soberish can be such a rewarding option to explore.

REASON #1: YOUR BASELINE WILL REGULATE ITSELF

When you stop drinking or cut back significantly, you give your body the opportunity to rebalance itself. Without the negative interference from alcohol, your central nervous system and endocrine system will begin to regulate themselves, leading to better moods and less intense emotions. Any feelings of anhedonia (see page 12) will begin to fade, and the connections and hobbies you hold so dear will start to bring you joy and pleasure once again. If your libido has been flagging, this too may improve. This process takes time, and there is no magic number, but using the tools in your soberish toolkit will help you to kickstart this process into high gear.

REASON #2: YOUR BRAIN CHEMISTRY WILL EVEN OUT

Because alcohol can penetrate our blood brain barrier (BBB), it is able to damage our brain by killing our brain cells and causing brain shrinkage. Thankfully, when you stop putting alcohol into your blood system, you give your brain time to heal and create new neural connections. During this time the brain can also regrow damaged tissue such as the grey and white matter that manage how we process information. Grey matter enables us to control our physical movement, memory and emotions.[36] Having the proper amount of functioning grey matter will allow you to gain more control over your emotional regulation, and you can strengthen the effect of this with the help of support groups, Cognitive Behavioural Therapy (CBT), mindfulness (see pages 160–71) and proper nutrition (see pages 97–113). Promising research on alcohol-induced brain damage shows rapid recovery of the brain from volume loss within the initial 14 days of abstinence,[37] offering hope to us all.

REASON #3: YOUR PHYSICAL APPEARANCE WILL IMPROVE

While I'm sure you are reading this book for deeper reasons than wrinkles, there's absolutely nothing wrong with wanting to look better – and you will. "Alcohol accelerates facial ageing similar to the way smoking does," explains Gillian Tietz.[38] Alcohol is a diuretic, and given that your skin is your largest organ, heavy consumption of alcohol can lead to dehydration, making your skin look shrivelled and dull. A 2019 study showed that those who were heavy drinkers, characterized by the consumption of eight or more drinks per week, were associated with increased wrinkles, under-eye puffiness, and midface volume loss.[39] Consumption of alcohol can cause nutrient depletion, which decreases your body's production of collagen, a protein in your body that maintains your skin's fullness and elasticity. Prevention is key with collagen, as repairing collagen loss is not as simple as taking supplements. However, research on human subjects is lacking in this area. Like collagen, your hair and nails need protein to grow strong and when you drink too much this can cause protein deficiency, leading to brittle nails, thinning hair and even hair loss. Drinking less also means healthier hair and nails. Alongside this, you can focus on consuming nutrients like iron, zinc, copper and protein to speed up the process.

REASON #4: YOU WILL GAIN MORE SELF-AWARENESS

With clearer cognition and higher brain functioning comes the ability to connect with yourself on a deeper level. In many ways, becoming more self-aware is the first step to higher personal growth. Self-awareness requires empathy, mindfulness and curiosity about who you really are as a person. I know that when I was drinking, I tended to be very self-centred. Not because I didn't care for those around me, but because I lacked the ability to think about others, which stopped me from being a good partner and friend in many situations. My drinking consumed me and left me completely unaware of my surroundings. By becoming more vulnerable and open in relationships and learning proper communication skills, I was able to let my guard down and share my emotions, which improved my connections with others. Self-awareness can also give you the ability to be a better decision-maker, empowering you to make choices that support your soberish lifestyle.

REASON #5: YOUR LIFE WILL BECOME MORE MANAGEABLE

When I was drinking it was as if I was on a never-ending apology tour. For years, I lived in a constant spiral of shame, which kept me in the cycle of drinking because I constantly felt overwhelmed and disappointed in my decision-making. I couldn't face my friends or family half of the time out of embarrassment, so I was reluctant to ask for help. When I finally let go of my ego and surrendered to the fact that I couldn't do this alone, things began to get better. When I first stopped drinking my problems didn't magically disappear, but I finally felt a sense of control, like I had the power to rebuild my life the way I intended to live it. I could rewrite my own narrative. It was as though a fog had lifted and I could see each situation and problem for what it really was, instead of the monsters I had made them out to be in my head from my constant anxiety. I prioritized what I needed to do, like go back to school, find a job I was passionate about and continue supporting my soberish lifestyle. I learned to be an essentialist, and let go of things that no longer served me, like unhealthy relationships, toxic friendships and focusing on what others thought of me. My anxiety began to lessen over time, as I was no longer afraid to look at my text messages from the night before, check my bank statement to look at my bar tab or apologize for the meaningless arguments I started. Life became less chaotic, and I holistically began to attract other people and opportunities that aligned with my new values and priorities. I stopped craving drama and started looking for stability. I kept people in my life who supported my new lifestyle and said adios to those who didn't. It's an indescribable feeling when you become "the reliable friend", the one others come to for advice, and you earn the trust back of those you love. Getting there is not a journey for the faint of heart, but I would do it all over again, knowing what's on the other side of all that hard work: true freedom.

These five reasons can have many other knock-on benefits in turn, such as being better able to cope with the demands of daily life, like work, study and managing finances, and enjoying improved health generally as your body's physical and mental systems begin to regulate themselves. If you do decide to cut back on drinking, you could be less prone to headaches and stomach upsets, sleep better (see pages 115–21) and even reduce the potential risk of developing a serious health condition such as certain types of cancer. Soberish grapevine member Katti H. puts it this way:

My booze-free benefits are various and vast. They overlap and also stand alone. These benefits have changed over time, yet continue to multiply. This life is fascinating and complex, yet also surprisingly simple and quiet at times.

Physically, I have more energy, incredible sleep, less anxiety, better sex and clearer skin.

Mentally, I am more present and grounded, less anxious and deeply connected to my inherent worth.

Spiritually, I know that the universe has my back, I'm connected to a source higher than myself, and I have released the constant internal war within.

The most impactful benefit is the clarity in my eyes now that I can finally meet my own gaze in the mirror. For years, I couldn't greet my own reflection because I knew I wasn't operating anywhere close to my highest potential.

My favourite benefit of my alcohol-free life is that I feel so much peace and alignment when my head hits the pillow each night (finally at a reasonable hour, ha!). I can honestly say that each day gets me closer to who I'm meant to be, and in many ways I'm already there.

CREATE YOUR OWN SOBERISH BENEFITS CHECKLIST

Thinking back to everything we've looked at so far, if you were to take a break or significantly cut back on your alcohol consumption, how might your life improve? Check off any of the answers that could pertain to you.

- [ ] Better mental health
- [ ] Improved performance at school or work
- [ ] Healthier romantic relationships
- [ ] More confidence
- [ ] Higher self-worth
- [ ] Saved money
- [ ] Improved immune system
- [ ] Deeper, more restful sleep
- [ ] Healthier skin and hair
- [ ] More energy
- [ ] Stronger libido
- [ ] Less stomach inflammation
- [ ] Significantly reduced risk of cancer
- [ ] Improved mood stability
- [ ] Deeper connections with loved ones

RECLAIM YOUR BRAIN!

You've got to the end of the first chapter and you're doing great! We've taken a look at the brain's dysfunctional relationship with alcohol, and seen how drinking can create neural pathways. Over time, these can lead all the way to destination AUD, but the good news is – thanks to the amazing neuroplasticity of the brain – we can rewire our grey matter and create new pathways that are way more fun and supportive.

We've also looked at the effect of alcohol on the brain in other ways, and how this can impact our health and behaviours, including why booze and mental health are not such a good match. And we saw how the diathesis–stress model of addiction can be helpful when it comes to understanding some key factors that may be shaping your own relationship with alcohol.

We've covered a lot of ground and identified a whole heap of issues and obstacles that we're potentially dealing with here. But, hey, anything that's worth having deserves a little work. There are so many benefits from creating a soberish lifestyle that suits you: you will look better! You will feel better! You will be able to think more clearly and, armed with the tools and information that I will be sharing with you in this book, make informed decisions that allow you to take control of your life. Ultimately, you will find the power to live your life the way you want to live it. So let's get started with taking back your narrative right now.

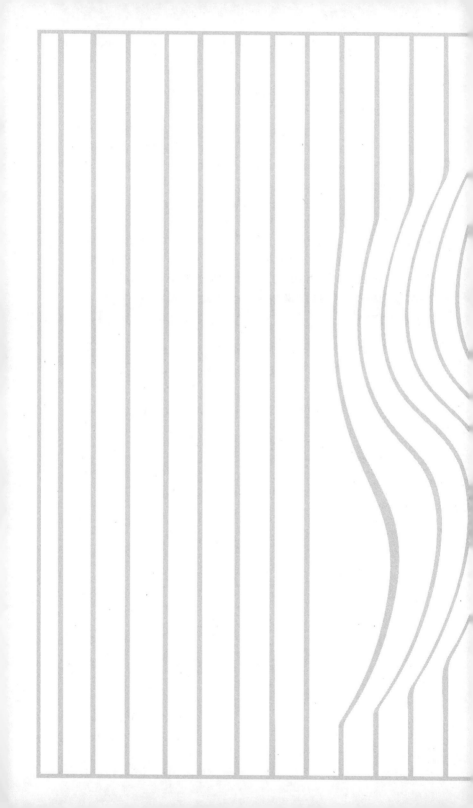

CHAPTER 2

Taking Back Your Narrative

Have you ever thought about the way you see and speak to yourself and noticed how this shapes the world around you? Ever since I can remember I've had a tendency to take a pessimistic outlook on life and I used to see the bad in everything. I'm sure I'm not alone in this feeling. Psychological research suggests that humans in general suffer from a negativity bias, which simply means we have a tendency to focus on the negative stimuli in our lives and dwell on past negative experiences.[1] This can be traced back to our evolution as human beings and how cave dwellers needed to be on the alert for constant danger. Back then, our ancestors were in literal life-or-death situations every day, so the more attentive they were to danger the more likely they were to survive. Those who did survive were the ones to procreate and pass on the genes that helped their offspring survive in turn. While I'm sure these traits were extremely helpful when it came to running from carnivorous animals and surviving with little shelter, the same traits are less helpful in today's Western world. Having our brains wired for constant negative stimuli in a civilized society impacts the way we think, respond and feel.

Another explanation for my pessimism can be attributed to the fact I have "negative affectivity", meaning a genetic tendency to experience more negative emotions. I read about this concept in *The Happiness Hypothesis* by Jonathan Haidt while on my quest to acquire a more positive mindset. I realized that while by nature I may be predisposed to a more negative outlook, especially as someone who has endured adversity, I can ultimately choose my own mindset through hard work and learned emotional intelligence.

For the longest time I was stuck in the vicious cycle of suffering, shame and self-loathing. I couldn't understand why all these horrible things were happening in my life, such as my parents' divorce, being sexually assaulted or the death of my best friend. I had a narrow view of the world and was poorly prepared to deal with any degree of grief or trauma. I had a serious lack of coping skills. It was no wonder I turned to pills and alcohol at a young age to try to regulate my emotions and get some sense of stability.

What I didn't realize at the time was that turning to things like alcohol, men and purging (you name it) was only pushing me further into the black hole I was trying to dig myself out of. I constantly flipped back and forth between the narrative of "poor me" and "wow, I'm disgusting". And trying to get out of that distorted thinking was impossible – or so I thought.

After I stopped drinking in 2016 I started to address all of the root issues of my problematic behaviour. It was as though my issues with alcohol were really a symptom of all of this underlying bad energy, which was growing inside of me and manifesting itself through binge drinking, eating disorders and other high-risk behaviours. Going alcohol-free for a long period allowed me to begin the process of regulating my emotions, healing and combatting my negative outlook on life. The best way I can describe it is it's like eroding your internal dam. Imagine all of the negative emotions, thought processes and life experiences you've ever had as these little prickly pear cactuses that get stuck inside of you. Over time they grow larger because we feed them through giving them validation with thoughts like, "I will always be like this," or, "I'm a bad person, I deserve to be treated this way." We may tend to avoid our problems altogether, thinking that by not talking about them they'll go away, but they don't. Eventually, all those prickly pear cactuses build up into a giant mass until we've created an internal dam where no emotions can move through us. This in turn causes mass dysregulation, which affects both our mental and physical states.

We drink so we don't feel the pain caused by our prickly pears, but all we are really doing is practising avoidance, which ultimately tends to increase our stress and anxiety. Negative emotions and traumas cannot be processed when we have alcohol in our system. Alcohol disrupts the balance of our hormones and important neurochemicals such as serotonin and dopamine which allow us to feel pleasure and happiness. It can also worsen our anxiety, depression and even cause suicidal thoughts. So while a booze-filled night out with our friends after being dumped seems like the solution, we're really just rubbing dirt into the wound.

The clear solution would be to remove the prickly pears from inside us, but in order to do this we have to address our problems – and who wants to do that? Clearly not us, because we've been using alcohol to avoid them in the first place. But the cringy truth of the matter is that *the only way out is through*. So in order to begin the process of healing and changing, we must face our uncomfortable emotions and pick out our prickly pears one by one.

THE POWER OF LANGUAGE

There is a famous quote from the Persian poet Hafiz that goes: "The words we speak become the house we live in." Nowhere is this truer than when it comes to changing your relationship with alcohol and finding the soberish lifestyle that suits you.

Having a positive perspective on a soberish lifestyle will not only make changing your relationship with alcohol easier, but it will make the experience empowering. When I first went into treatment in 2015, there really wasn't much available in the way of positive programmes or support groups. I was taught my drinking was a life or death situation and that I needed to be anonymous in my journey. While that may be true for some, it wasn't the message I needed to hear and it most definitely didn't help me quit. While I did get sober through the 12-Step programmes, it wasn't their fear tactics that helped me build a foundation; it was the accountability of the programme, being of service to others and the large young sober people's community in Los Angeles. I would walk into young people's (YP) meetings and see girls who made being sober look so cool. It was like I'd entered an alternate reality where being on drugs made you the outcast and being "clean and sober" made you part of the in-crowd. Instead of feeling like a fuck-up, this group made me feel empowered about my choice to stop drinking, like we had figured out some incredible secret to the universe that only we knew about. I felt part of something, and I had never felt that way before.

When I left the programme, trying to find that sense of community was the hardest part, which is why I created my first online community (1,000 Hours Dry, aka The Dry Club). Again, this was before sober/ish/curious Instagram became large and welcoming, so the whole experience was terrifying. I was going against everything I'd been taught, but I knew there were other people out there like me, who wanted a different lifestyle but who didn't want to conform to traditional programming. I realized quickly how many people there were who were looking for help but who didn't want to identify as an alcoholic or step into a meeting, so I tried changing the language to be more inclusive around the process and it instantly became more inviting. I had never realized how impactful the language we use can be on our mindset and the way we view the world until I started to learn more and shift to a more positive perspective.

According to sociologist Howard Becker's Labelling Theory, which he described in his 1963 book *Outsiders*, once you have been labelled a "deviant" (i.e., someone who behaves outside of cultural norms), you begin to face a new set of problems that stem from self-judgement and stereotypes.[2] Let's say you label yourself an alcoholic: according to Becker, that label will attach you to a number of negative connotations and stereotypical characteristic traits associated with anyone else bearing the label.[3] Now others begin to see you as how they perceive an alcoholic to be, versus who you are as a person. The label then becomes your identity, whether or not you like it: "*Oh, did you hear about Kayla? Apparently she's an alcoholic? She must have some serious issues, I don't think I can trust her to pick up my kids from school anymore.*" A nasty generalization, but the ugly truth is that a lot of people think this way and it goes far beyond those of us who struggle with alcohol. Stereotypes go deep into race, gender, culture and religion, fuelled by misinformation and ignorance. And the most hurtful part is how untrue most stereotypes are, especially when it comes to those of us who struggle with alcohol. However, because our general behaviour falls outside "cultural norms", we too are faced with these issues.

Self-judgement and the perpetuation of a negative view of self can also be a major problem when we label ourselves – and as if in a never-ending cycle, the way we label ourselves can often be based on how others treat us. Sociologist Charles Cooley's "Looking-Glass Theory" states that our perception of ourselves is based on how others see us. We measure our value based on the judgements of others, which forms our self-concept.

Have you ever considered how others see you? Perhaps your parents, your partner or your friends? I absolutely think about this, more than I'd care to admit. *"What will this outfit say about me?" "How will this Instagram post be received? Is it too controversial?" "Maybe I should sneak this third glass of wine so no one sees."* It's a harsh reality, but the world we currently live in is very much based on external appearances and how others perceive us. Social media is a perfect example. We've created an entire world where everything is designed to impress others and create a sense of external gratification – but none of it is even real.

HOW TO DISRUPT NEGATIVE THINKING PATTERNS

Labelling can be so problematic when it comes to understanding who we really are. If the label has connotations or is stigmatic, then we are at risk of coming to believe those negative views are true. In the same way, we may begin to believe the negative beliefs of others when they repeatedly say hurtful things to us like, "You aren't good enough," or, "You aren't thin enough." We risk taking on the connotations of the negative stereotypes of our own labels: "alcoholic", "addict", "drunk", "lush". If I tell myself I am an alcoholic, over and over, and that I will never be able to stop drinking, am I not more likely to accept this as truth and continue to drink? And if I am sober, but I'm told that if I slip up and drink I will almost certainly end up right back where I started, am I not more likely to go into a full-blown relapse if a slip happens to occur? It's a self-fulfilling prophecy. So how do we stop ourselves from influencing our own goals and futures in a negative way? We change our narrative. We take our power back and we choose positive language that encourages us to flourish and grow. I'll give you some examples of unhelpful, stigmatic types of label versus some empowering and inclusive alternatives:

STIGMATIC LABEL

- **Alcoholic/addict:** Has a negative connotation, and is viewed as incorrect in terms of current medical terminology.
- **Sobriety:** Associated with those in recovery from an AUD.
- **Alcohol abuse:** The term "abuse" was found to have a high association with negative judgements.[4]
- **Relapse:** Implies a "full-blown" return to old drinking behaviours.

EMPOWERING AND INCLUSIVE ALTERNATIVE TERMINOLOGY

- **Alcohol use disorder**: Proper terminology used by the DSM-5 and ICD-10, which allows for the existence of a spectrum ranging from mild to severe.
- **Alcohol-free:** Can be used by anyone choosing to live an alcohol-free lifestyle.
- **Alcohol misuse:** Implies a problem without stigmatizing the individual.
- **Backslide/fall-forward**: Can be a slip, or short lapse of judgement where one drinks on an occasion, but it does not change the course of the individual's soberish journey.

I want to be clear that how you choose to identify is your decision, and there is no right or wrong way. If giving yourself a label feels empowering or helps keep you accountable, then I encourage you to continue doing what works for you. When I started my journey I identified as an "alcoholic/addict," then "recovered alcoholic/addict," then "sober"; and now, based on my belief in the power of positive language, I choose simply to say I live a *soberish lifestyle*. Soberish can be a label or a lifestyle: what's most important is that it signifies you have taken back your power from alcohol.

WHAT WORDS DO YOU USE?

What sort of language do you use around alcohol and drinking? Judgemental or jokey? Serious or free and easy? Have you ever stopped to think about the narrative(s) that you may be telling yourself through the vocabulary you use? Take a moment now to consider this . . .

★ First, write down all of the words and phrases you associate with alcohol and with the wide range of people who drink it, including yourself.

★ Now I want you to take a moment to think carefully about each of your responses. Are they in any way judgemental? Is the tone negative, positive or neutral? Do they compartmentalize different types of drinkers and drinking?

★ Reflect on your findings. Do you find you sway more on the side of stigmatic or inclusive terminology, as described above?

Keeping this awareness in mind, take a moment now to think about how and why you use the language you do around alcohol. Perhaps you know someone in your life who struggles with their relationship with alcohol and you have had negative experiences that may have coloured your view? Or maybe your list of positive associations is longer? How central is alcohol to your experiences? Why do you think you use the language around drink and drinking in the ways that you do?

CULTIVATE SELF-AWARENESS

How you speak about yourself helps to shape your world, in terms of your self-belief and the ways in which other people see you. The good news is that while some of us may be naturally inclined toward a more negative mindset, with a bit of hard work, dedication and awareness, we can start to change this from the outside in by reframing the language we use about ourselves. In this way, we can begin to reclaim our narrative and get to work on those toxic emotions that build up inside us, which we likely have been trying to avoid through drinking.

As part of your soberish journey, it's time now to start to get to know yourself properly. This isn't about beating yourself up, taking yourself to task or throwing yourself a pity party, but about starting to think about your behaviours around booze with honesty and without judgement. Keep an open mind and be prepared for some surprises along the way.

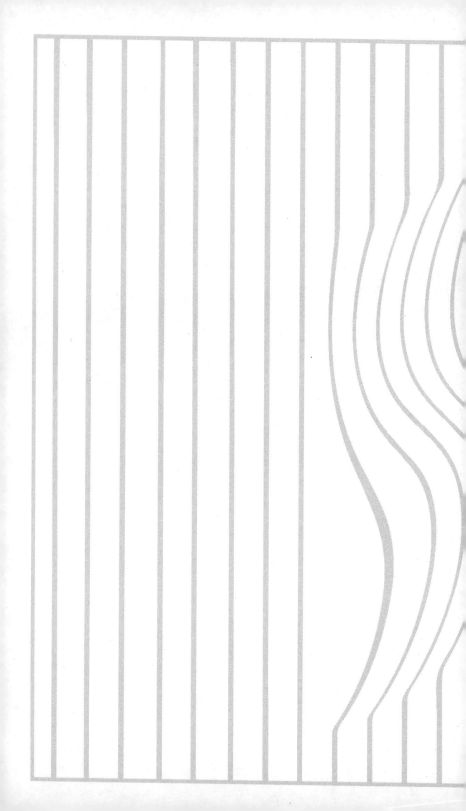

CHAPTER 3

Finding
Answers
Through
Introspection

Before we can spring into action and make big changes, we'll need to figure out the role alcohol plays in our lives. Are we social drinkers? Emotional drinkers? Maybe we understand at a surface level that drinking isn't helping us reach our goals or is hazardous to our relationships, but we continue to do the same thing anyways, hoping for different results. If this sounds like you, you're not alone, which is why I've come up with a self-assessment exercise to guide you to the root of your drinking habits. Once we find the root, we can address it and make some tangible, positive changes.

WHY DO YOU THINK YOU DRINK?

Have you ever questioned why you really drink, or what happens when you do? Obvious answers may come to mind, like "because that's what my friends and I do", "because it's fun", or, "because it's an easy way to relax" . . . We may turn to alcohol for a whole heap of other reasons too, such as using it as a social lubricant to handle social anxiety or shyness, for stress reduction, as a coping mechanism or reward (the "treat" at the end of a long day), or even a form of self-care if, for example, we try to self-medicate with it or use it as a way to cope with loneliness or boredom.

In the next exercise, I'd like you to start thinking a little more deeply about any reasons that apply to you. Again, there're no right or wrong answers here. Just answer from your gut.

WHAT KIND OF DRINKER AM I?

When do you usually find yourself drinking, and what happens when you do? Circle the answer(s) below that resonate with you the most, and then turn to the "If you answered" section on page 51, where you will find a key that explains what your answers suggest about your drinking habits. You will also discover insights from the soberish community, describing how these sorts of behaviours manifested themselves in their own lives.

① When I drink, I . . .

a. tend to stick to my limit or I don't drink.
b. often do so after a demanding or emotional situation.
c. usually drink four or more drinks on one occasion.
d. tend to black out and get into high-risk situations like fights or drinking and driving.
e. usually do so on an empty stomach.
f. like to pair it with my food or experience tastings.
g. don't think too much about it, it's just something to do.
h. try to decompress.

② I drink so that I . . .

a. can enjoy time hanging out with friends or at an event.
b. don't have to feel my anxiety, depression or other heavy emotions.
c. can get drunk.

   d.   can feel better about myself, the way I look
        or how I feel about my weight.
   e.   feel like I'm tapping into a kind of life energy
        – but I'm careful to offset the calories.
   f.   can enjoy my meal more and have a sensory
        experience.
   g.   don't have to be so bored.
   h.   can let go of stress.

③ **I drink to get drunk . . .**

   a.   never.
   b.   and not deal with my feelings or mental health
        issues.
   c.   most of the time.
   d.   because that's what I do.
   e.   because my reward is to get drunk more quickly
        if I don't eat too much.
   f.   unintentionally sometimes, when it feels like
        you can't have too much of a good thing.
   g.   if there's nothing much else to do.
   h.   to release the build-up of tension.

④ **When I drink . . .**

   a.   I usually do so with friends or at an event but
        rarely if ever alone.
   b.   I do so after something has triggered an
        uncomfortable emotion that I don't want to feel.
   c.   it's hard for me to stick to my limits. I usually
        drink more than I plan to. I have tried putting
        rules around my drinking in the past but haven't
        been able to stick to them.
   d.   I can get myself into high-risk situations like
        blacking out, fights, unprotected sex, getting
        arrested or hospitalized.

e. I tend to get intoxicated quickly because I don't eat before I drink, or I purge what I eat while I'm drinking to stay drunk.

f. it's usually for the purpose of enhancing my meal or my overall experience of an event.

g. it's usually to fill the time, or it's just something "to do" with friends.

h. it's like I'm off-duty and no longer have to take responsibility for everything.

⑤ **People in my life have expressed concern for my drinking . . .**

a. not in my experience.

b. yes, they worry about my mental health and wellbeing.

c. yes, I've been told I drink too much.

d. yes, my loved ones are concerned for my health and safety because of my drinking.

e. yes, they worry I do not eat enough so that I can save my calories for alcohol.

f. never to me.

g. not that I'm aware of.

h. sometimes, but mostly they appreciate it's a case of "work hard, play hard".

If you answered:

★ "a" to most questions you may be a social drinker. Social drinker Leah A said: "Drinking for me has been something to do with friends and a way to connect with others."

★ "b" to most questions you may be a self-medicating drinker. Ashley M. put it this way: "I was drinking huge amounts every night to try to avoid coping with a sexual assault and abusive relationship. It helped, until it didn't."

★ **"c"** or **"d"** to most questions you may be a binge or high-risk drinker. Andy Z. described the compulsion to binge-drink: "I could rarely – if ever – have only one beer. One became 4, 5, 12 pretty quickly." Emily M. explained how risky this behaviour can be: "After college I was sort of discovering myself and often found myself needing to get drunk before getting intimate, or sometimes getting too drunk to the point of sexual assault, unbeknownst to me"; while Madison J. revealed how high-risk drinking can literally be life-threatening: "I got into my first bar fight at 16. I've been kicked out of more bars than I can count. Missed countless days of work due to hangovers. It wasn't until two hospitalizations in 2021 that I finally decided to try and get sober."

★ **"e"** to most questions you may be a "drunkorexic". Steph S. explained what this looked like for her: "Restricting during the week or only eating 'healthy' foods in preparation for the weekend, working out excessively the night after drinking to "burn off" the alcohol and calories, being secretly excited about vomiting from alcohol because it meant the alcohol and food was leaving my system."

★ **"f"** to most questions you may be a sensory drinker. As Thea F. put it: "I don't enjoy being drunk. I do like a slight buzz to help loosen conversation and put myself at ease. But pairing with foods, cheeses, meats, fish, pasta, etc. is always a more enjoyable experience."

★ **"g"** to most questions you may be a boredom drinker. Nikita described how this type of drinking can creep up on us: "I started noticing drinking for no real reason, but very often. I thought you only had a problem with alcohol use if you abused it, i.e. binge or stress drinking."

★ **"h"** to most questions you may be a stress drinker. H. H. describes the urge to drink as a way to unwind after a work trip: "I remember so often I would call my boyfriend on the way home from a trip and ask if we had alcohol at home. If I was getting home late, I made sure to call the night before. I couldn't fathom the idea of ending a work trip without a drink to come home to."

Write down the results of your drinker archetype, based on your answers. (There can be more than one.) Why do you feel that category or those categories best describe your drinking? What influences you to drink? (This could be anything – from peer pressure, FOMO, the music you listen to and the shows you watch, to stress or social anxiety, even your culture or your environment.) I'd like you to keep your answers in mind as we progress through this book.

• •

THE DIFFERENT TYPES OF DRINKING

Even if you don't think that some, or any, of the drinking archetypes apply to you, it's a good idea to be able to recognize them as you set out on your soberish journey. There may be changing circumstances in all our lives that could get us reaching for the bottle for any number of different reasons. That's why I'd suggest you familiarize yourself with all the archetypes as well as any that seem to fit you best at the moment.

THE SOCIAL DRINKER

"I don't crave alcohol at home or by myself. I can do without drinking and go to dinner without needing or wanting an alcoholic beverage. I don't love the taste of it a lot of the time."
Leah A.

You like to drink while hanging out with friends or at events. Your drinking doesn't tend to disrupt your life in a negative way — that is, unless you hang out with your friends quite a lot, have to drink with work clients regularly or tend to experience social anxiety. Like Brooke L., you automatically associate going out with drinking:

I started drinking because it represented independence, 'coolness' and adulthood. Growing up in the US, you aspired to be a young adolescent. Late teen years are featured in most films and TV shows as the 'time of your life', and college culture in the South is heavily reliant on drinking. Drinking was the default mode of socializing and I loved meeting people and networking. So from age 13 to 23 I was a social drinker, with my alcohol intake widely ranging based on my access to it, my pressures and influences and my overall environment.

For you, drinking at home isn't necessarily appealing, but nor is attending events that don't have alcohol. As we've seen, the definition of low-risk drinking differs by country, but the overall consensus seems to be no more than 14 drinks a week across the board.[1] If you find yourself drinking more than what is considered to be moderate drinking, or you also circled a lot of "C"s and "D"s in the quiz, you may be more than just a social drinker.

THE SELF-MEDICATING DRINKER

> "It started with drinking to dull feelings about certain events and situations, which ultimately hushed my true self enough that I didn't make the changes I desperately needed to make. Which led to drinking to numb an increasing number of events, relationships, and situations. It got to the point that I was drinking nearly all the time, to escape a life that was entirely wrong for me and built on what others wanted and who I felt I had to be in order to be loved and accepted."
> **Nedda H.**

When we have experienced Adverse Childhood Experiences (ACE) such as home-life dysfunction, abuse, neglect or other significant traumas, we are at higher risk of turning to alcohol to self-medicate. (If you or anyone you know has experienced sexual assault or domestic abuse, please turn to page 288 for resources.) Those with a high level of ACE are also more likely to develop other emotional disorders such as depression, anger-management issues, anxiety or self-harming compulsions. The combination of these disorders and a lack of coping mechanisms can lead to later-life issues such as unhealthy relationships, loss of jobs, run-ins with the law and alcohol dependency.

While alcohol can make us feel temporarily happy or disassociated from our negative feelings, it ultimately leads to worsening symptoms of stress, anxiety and depression. The cycle of self-medication is vicious, because we drink to feel relief but eventually dig ourselves deeper into the problem.

I would consider myself a former self-medicator, among other drinking archetypes. One of the major reasons I drank was to deal with the anxiety and panic attacks I was experiencing from untreated OCD and Panic Disorder. I also experienced a lot of instability in my adolescence, as a child of multiple divorces, moving every two to four years because of my parents' jobs and an unhealthy household environment. For me, the combination of undiagnosed mental health disorders and an unstable childhood was a recipe for alcohol and substance misuse disorders, along with other disorders such as eating disorders and body dysmorphia. The power I find in this archetype is that so many strong, inspiring people come from similar backgrounds, which reminds me that my past and where I come from do not define my future.

THE BINGE DRINKER

"My drinking definitely started with me wanting to fit in. I didn't know my tolerance was low back then and I was prone to blacking out. I resented the fact I couldn't drink like 'normal people' and not black out all the time."
Alyssa B.

According to the National Institute of Alcohol Abuse and Alcoholism (NIAAA), binge drinking is considered drinking more than four drinks for women and five drinks for men on any one occasion, usually within the space of two hours.[2] Binge drinking can lead to serious health problems and high-risk behaviours, including alcohol abuse and dependence, driving under the influence, sexual assault, domestic violence and murder. It can also result in chronic diseases such as cirrhosis, pancreatitis, various cancers, high blood pressure and psychological problems. Research indicates excessive binge drinking during the adolescent period can alter the trajectory of brain development and cause lingering deficits in social, attention, memory and other cognitive functions.[3]

I would definitely have considered myself a binge drinker when I was actively consuming. Once I had the first drink, all bets were off. I could rarely control my intake and one drink quickly became five or six, which was especially dangerous considering it led me to high-risk behaviours. Even though I didn't necessarily drink every day, I easily went over the weekly recommended limit of 14 in two nights minimum. I was by no means drinking to enjoy the taste or to create an ambiance, I was drinking to get drunk. Period.

THE HIGH-RISK DRINKER

"My life was constantly in shambles. Even if I tried to cut down, I mentally and physically could not. I would wake up shaking or in jail cells; every morning I would check my car bumper for blood because I didn't remember getting home. I lost my children, my marriage, my family and my freedom because of my drinking."
Cassady V.

Similar to the binge drinker, the high-risk drinker continues to drink at heavy levels despite negative consequences. High-risk drinking is defined as four or more drinks per day or 14 per week for men, and three or more drinks a day or seven per week for women.[4] If you've ever been on academic probation, kicked out of a bar, cheated on a partner, or been arrested or hospitalized due to your drinking, you may fit into this category. I use these examples because I have experienced them all, more than once, because of my drinking. Nothing could have stopped the cycle I was in until I was really willing to recognize that alcohol was the problem, not the solution. High-risk drinking can have some sobering consequences, as Nikita M. explains:

> I woke up in a hospital with a doctor telling me, "You are 34 years old, you came in with a .54 BAC and I can't get your blood pressure down. I am pretty sure you are about to have a stroke. I called your father, he should get to say goodbye. My nurses shouldn't have to see this." And then he walked out. That was the last time I ever drank.

If you believe this category fits you, the fact that you are here reading this book demonstrates that you've taken a massive step toward awareness and change, and I want you to know that no matter where you are on your journey, that means something.

"DRUNKOREXIA" OR ALCOHOL ANOREXIA

"In college I struggled with orthorexia (obsessing over being "healthy" to an unhealthy degree). I also binge-drank every weekend which was not healthy and therefore went directly against my orthorexic tendencies and beliefs. I felt so guilty after weekends of binge drinking and eating 'bad' foods that

I would overcompensate with restriction
and over-exercise during the week, only
to repeat the cycle the next weekend."
Steph S.

The word "drunkorexic" is a non-medical term that refers to someone who restricts their eating so that they can "save" the calories for drinking, or who purges their alcohol after they have experienced its intoxicating effects. In addition to developing a serious eating disorder, there are other dangers that come with drinking on an empty stomach, such as higher blood alcohol levels, stronger chance of intoxication or blacking out, gastritis and eventually stomach cancer.[5] According to addiction specialist Dr Susanne Reed, there is a 41 per cent comorbidity rate among people with eating disorders and addiction. Research also indicates that those with bulimia nervosa are twice as likely to misuse alcohol than individuals with other eating disorders.[6]

THE SENSORY DRINKER

The sensory drinker prefers to drink as an experience, not necessarily for the intoxicating effects. They enjoy the different aromas and tastes, and take pride in being able to pair their meals well with their drinks. They see alcohol as a way to enhance a meal and enjoy activities such as wine tasting.

Thea F. describes this attitude:

I mostly drink socially, but I enjoy cooking for friends, and having good wine pairings as an enjoyable and fun experience. I do enjoy feeling slightly looser when around company, but never drink so much as I become impaired because that isn't the point. I got into this because I started with coffee and tea pairings and it is a natural extension.

THE BOREDOM DRINKER

> "It starts out so small it's hard to even notice, but looking back over the last few years I can see how it escalated quickly. Not having any awareness of the unhealthy aspects of alcohol was the underlying issue."
> **Nikya V.**

If this is you, you tend to drink the most when you are bored. Even if you don't particularly love alcohol or its effects, for whatever reason you find yourself reaching for a drink when you have nothing to do. Perhaps you find yourself drinking mindlessly in the evening while watching Netflix, at home when you've finished all your chores around the house or on the weekend when you don't have plans. You may have noticed an escalation in how much or how often you were drinking during Covid lockdown, when everything was shut down, and now you're looking to kick the habit before it becomes problematic.

Drinking out of boredom is quite real and it can turn quickly into problematic drinking if you aren't swift to notice your behaviour. I have been guilty of this kind of drinking in the past, particularly when I was living with family after my separation. I was thousands of miles away from my home, my support system and my community. I went from living in a city by the beach where the weather is always beautiful, with a plethora of different restaurants, social activities and my soberish support system, to staying in a very small town in the Midwest, where I knew no one and the only thing to do outside of exercise was watch football. I went from someone who gave myself permission to drink mindfully once or twice a year, to someone who was drinking once a week out of sheer boredom. I was extremely lonely and I noticed alcohol was one of my only ways to connect with the friends I made and with the dates I went on, because we didn't seem to have a lot else in common. In hindsight, it wasn't an excuse, but it was an observation that reminded me of the importance of support and human connection. If you're someone in a small town and this hits close to home, I understand your frustration. When the culture of where you live is rooted in alcohol or activities that revolve around drinking it can be extremely difficult to break the mould and go out on your own. Finding online support and exploring new hobbies can be an effective way to combat boredom. You never know who you'll meet while partaking in non-alcohol related activities like hiking, running, gaming or book clubs.

THE STRESS DRINKER

"It's an easy way to take a load off, get to know your co-workers in a casual setting, and decompress. I got so used to having a drink at the end of my day that eventually I didn't know how to decompress without one. Long day? Drink. Mean passengers? Drink. Cranky crew? Drink. Day off? Drink."
H. H.

We all experience stress, but some of us tend to reach for a drink whenever we experience hardships instead of using healthier coping mechanisms. A recent study from the NIAAA found that those who experience higher levels of stress tend to drink more.[7] Using alcohol to deal with uncomfortable or painful emotions can point to the development of long-term alcohol problems such as alcohol use disorder. It's important to find alternative ways to deal with stress and to eliminate our non-essential stressors to increase our overall wellbeing.

The four main causes of stress that can lead to heavy drinking include:[8]

- ★ **General life stress:** moving house, divorce, starting a new job, starting your freshman year of college.
- ★ **Catastrophic life events:** terrorist attack, pandemic, natural disaster.
- ★ **Childhood stress:** physical, emotional or sexual abuse, neglect.
- ★ **Ethnic minority stress:** experiencing prejudice, being the victim of a hate crime, being overlooked for a promotion.

Kristi G. described how stress contributed to her overuse of alcohol in her free time:

> *I was high-functioning and didn't let my drinking affect my work; I received accolades and praise, and then quietly binged on the weekend, wasting all my time off being drunk and messy or recovering from being drunk and messy.*

Now you've learned more about them, how do these descriptions sit with you? Do any of them ring especially true or make you feel uncomfortable, or even angry or upset? That's OK. Just give yourself some time to process how you're feeling. A lot of this stuff can be challenging to deal with, especially at first, but it gets easier, I promise.

This chapter is all about beginning to develop self-awareness, a kind of everyday mindfulness that will make it easier for you to make sense of why you do the things you do when it comes to drinking. And that in turn will give you more power over the choices you make. Which brings us on to some great practices to help with this.

CREATIVE SOUL-SEARCHING

Introspection doesn't have to mean hours of navel-gazing or, at the other extreme, taking a long look in the mirror and then beating yourself up because you don't like what you see. Here are three simple and effective ways to get to know more about what drives your drinking patterns.

•••••••••••••••••••••••••••••••••••••

CREATE A BOOZE BOARD

A vision board is a collage of images and words that represent somebody's dreams and goals. A booze board is not about attracting more alcohol into your life (!) but getting a clearer picture of your attitude toward it.

You will need:
a piece of blank paper or a poster board
a selection of magazines
additional images and words sourced from artworks,
    books, photos or printouts (optional)
scissors
a glue stick
pens, markers or other drawing utensils

★ Consider what terms and emotions you
    associate with the word "alcohol". Now, go
    through the magazines and cut out any words

or images that illustrate this. You can draw, write or print these out too.

★ Stick your cut-out words and images onto the paper or board in a way that expresses the way alcohol currently makes you feel.

★ Unlike a vision board, which you would leave in a place where you can see it, once you've completed your booze board, take a moment to reflect on it and then put it away.

★ Come back to this board in two weeks' time, then again in four weeks and compare your emotions and associations. Have they changed?

. . . .

DIG DEEP

In Part Two of this book, I'm going to be sharing some tools that have helped me personally, one of which is mindfulness. A very important part of my own mindfulness practice involves visualization. If you're not familiar with the concept, visualization is a type of meditation in which you use guided imagery or mental images to obtain a goal like a specific state of mind or for problem-solving. I personally use visualization to reduce my anxiety, declutter my mind, set goals and process negative emotions. In this exercise we'll be using guided imagery to evaluate your current drinking habits so that you have a better understanding of your relationship with alcohol. Start by reading the prompts below, then follow the guidelines to complete the exercise.

★ Before we begin, I want you to find a quiet place where you can sit or lie down without being disturbed. Find a pen and paper and take this into the space with you. Then turn off your phone and shut the door. With the pen and paper at your side, make sure you are sitting or lying down in a comfortable position that makes you feel relaxed.

★ Once you are comfortable, focus on your breathing. Take a deep breath in for four counts, hold for four counts and release for four counts. Repeat this breathing exercise a few times until you feel your shoulders begin to relax, your jaw begin to loosen and your heart rate begin to slow down.

★ Once you feel grounded, close your eyes and picture the last time you had a negative drinking experience. Think about that day in detail. What led up to your drinking? Were you perhaps triggered by a certain person, the time of day or a stressful situation? Consider why you decided to drink; maybe you were hoping to relieve yourself of an uncomfortable emotion, reward yourself for a hard day or were attending a social event?

★ How did you feel after that first drink? Were you relieved, or anxious for another? After you started drinking, what happened? What led up to the events that turned the situation into a negative experience? Did something occur that would not have happened had you not drank? Replay the negative experience to identify where things shifted.

★ After the negative event or situation transpired, what happened? Did you continue to drink or was this event a "wake-up call" to stop consuming? Ask yourself how you felt the next day about your negative experience. When you woke up, were you familiar with your surroundings? Hungover? Unable to recall all or any of the prior day or night's events? How did you feel?

★ Now before we leave this visualization I want you to remember that this last experience, and any that came before it, does not define you. You are worthy of change, forgiveness, love and evolution. Repeat to yourself, "I am worthy, I am loved, I am changing." Continue to repeat these mantras as you get back into your body.

★ Wiggle your toes and fingers. Begin to feel all the sensations in your body. Awaken each part by moving before returning to your breath.

★ Complete this visualization by taking a deep breath in for four counts, hold for four counts and release for four counts. Continue this breathing exercise until you feel yourself back in the present moment.

★ Open your eyes, take out your pen and paper, and write down what you saw. Do so without thinking, worrying about grammar or legibility – this is called free writing. When you are done recalling your visualization, answer the following four questions:

1. How did this experience change the way I view my relationship with alcohol?

2. How can I use this experience and any other negative event involving my alcohol consumption to strengthen my decision to change my relationship with alcohol?

3. How can I move forward, starting today, with self-compassion for the version of me I feel shame toward?

4. If a similar situation happens that triggers me to want to drink, how can I handle it without doing so?

PHONE A FRIEND

Sometimes the people around us can notice our behaviour or demeanour change when we don't. When we are under the influence of alcohol, we lack self-awareness and may be acting out of character without even noticing. Getting an outside perspective can help us see the whole picture more clearly.

★ Speak to a few friends or loved ones who have been around you while you have been under the influence and ask them how you behaved. Did your personality change at all? Did you tend to be more impulsive or put yourself into risky situations? Has your friend or loved one ever been concerned about your drinking? Ask these questions with an open mind and without judgement of the answers or yourself.

★ If you speak with more than one person, look for patterns in their answers and then reflect on them. How did their answers make you feel? Did their answers validate your own concerns or fears about your relationship with alcohol? How can you use these answers to further motivate your desire to change?

HARNESSING THE POWER OF SELF-AWARENESS

Self-awareness can act like a secret super-power and allow us to control our actions, develop a sense of perspective and influence the outcomes we want to achieve in our lives. This is why it's important to recognize even those emotions that are difficult to acknowledge, instead of attempting to drown them in a vat of booze. The exercises in this chapter have been designed to give you a little more insight into your relationship with alcohol, so that you can draw on your own self-awareness as you take the next steps on your soberish journey and start setting yourself some goals to work toward.

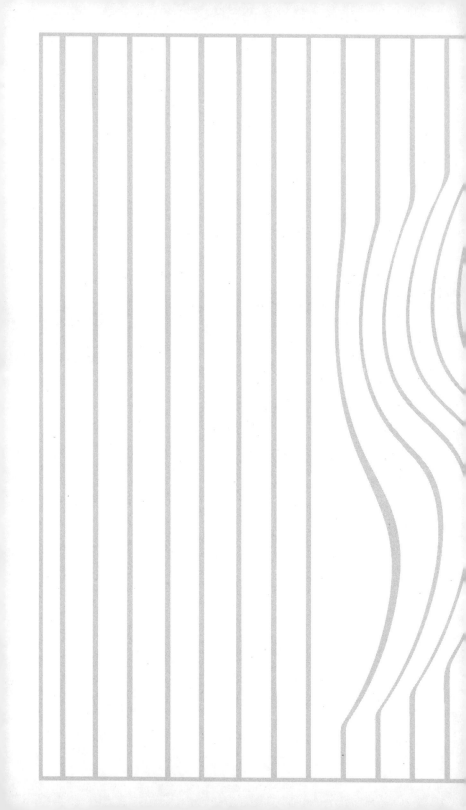

CHAPTER 4

The Keys to Success: Goal-Setting and Preparation

Understanding why and how you got to a point where alcohol was no longer serving you in a positive way is a foundational step in creating the soberish lifestyle you desire. Now that you have identified the way in which you drink, you can gain a better understanding of how you can change your pattern of behaviour. Through your self-assessment you gained awareness and a deeper understanding of the role alcohol plays in your life. Having gained this insight, you can begin to look at what needs to change and set yourself some new goals to aim toward instead.

By creating a Plan of Action, you can create a new set of habits to replace the old ones that were negatively impacting your wellbeing, and have a range of tools to draw upon when you need them. This is the second step in the pioneering psychologist Kurt Lewin's model of change, a social psychology theory which helps us to understand the stages of change in a more digestible way.[1] Lewin's model explains that change is like an ice cube: in order for you to get to where you want, you must first "unfreeze" the ice cube, which represents recognizing and identifying what needs to change (which you did in chapter 3 through your self-assessment). Then in the second phase – "change" – you begin to plan and implement the lifestyle and behavioural changes you want to make and set goals that reflect the life you want to attain, which we are going to do next. Lastly, you freeze the ice cube by integrating the changes you've made into your everyday life, stabilizing your new habits and developing ways to sustain your success. All of which we will discuss in later chapters. For now, let us focus on the second stage.

DESIGN THE LIFE YOU WANT

One of the top reasons we fall back into old habits, or drink even after we said we weren't going to, is because we still hold drinking at a higher value at that moment than our sobriety or cutback journey. This usually happens when we are stressed, overwhelmed or anxious and we get a case of the "fuck-its". For whatever reason, at that moment, drinking alcohol becomes more valuable to us than our desire not to drink and everything else goes out the window.

Sound familiar? Having a strong toolkit to hand can help you avoid these moments, but even more important is setting future goals that keep your eyes on the prize. When your future priorities trump your desire to drink, no matter how stressful the situation, you have the strongest armour you could ask for.

One of my favourite goal-setting techniques is called "SMART goals", developed by George Doran, Arthur Miller and James Cunningham in their 1981 article "There's a S.M.A.R.T. Way to Write Management Goals and Objectives".[2] The reason I like this technique so much is its simplicity. The acronym SMART stands for:[3]

- ★ **Specific:** Objective clearly states, so anyone reading it can understand, what will be done and who will do it.
- ★ **Measurable:** Objective includes how the action will be measured. Measuring your objectives helps you determine if you are making progress. This keeps you on track and on schedule.
- ★ **Achievable:** Objective is realistic given the realities faced in the community. Setting reasonable objectives helps set up the project for success.

- ★ **Relevant:** A relevant objective makes sense; that is, it fits the required purpose, the culture and structure of the community, and it addresses the vision of the project.
- ★ **Time-bound:** Every objective has a specific timeline for completion.

Having goals gives us something to work toward and focus on. They push us forward and give us a constant reminder we are on our way to becoming a higher version of ourselves. When we prioritize and value our future over drinking, we create a lifestyle over which alcohol no longer has power. In those "fuck-it" moments, instead of picking up a drink, you can now think about all of the goals you have set up for yourself and decide what is more important. You'll begin to notice that once you start setting goals, alcohol only inhibits your ability to reach them, which makes drinking less attractive. Below is a list of different kinds of goals you can set for yourself to strengthen your new lifestyle:

- ★ **Personal:** For example, would you like to have a better sleep schedule, cut down on screen time and read more books, or explore a hobby that interests you?
- ★ **Professional:** Have you been trying to manifest a promotion, but have yet to take the next steps to get there? Have you always wanted to branch out and start your own business?
- ★ **Physical:** It's common knowledge that alcohol can have a serious impact on your physical health, so what would you like to improve physically about yourself while re-evaluating your relationship with alcohol? Maybe you have envisioned yourself crossing the finish

line at a half marathon, or perhaps you've always wanted to have clearer skin?

★ **Emotional:** Alcohol is not only detrimental to our physical health, it can take a toll on our mental health and emotional wellbeing. Do you have goals of becoming happier or more emotionally stable? If so, is therapy or meditation something you would like to try?

★ **Interpersonal:** This is the ideal opportunity to begin working on mending or strengthening your relationships with your family, friends, peers and co-workers, etc. Perhaps you want to meet more like-minded individuals by starting or joining a book club, or finally make amends with your sibling? There's no time like the present.

★ **Financial:** Alcohol can impact both our brain and our wallet in negative ways. As we rebuild strength in our prefrontal cortex, we also begin repairing our decision-making skills. For many, this helps with financial issues: when we have improved decision-making ability and impulse control, we can focus on managing our spending. Not to mention all of the money you'll save on booze, Ubers, late-night munchies and replacing lost phones!

CREATE YOUR OWN SMART GOALS

One of my favourite goal-setting exercises involves focusing on the following three types: personal, financial and professional goals. I want you to create a list of your own goals in each of these categories.

★ Reflect on what you want to achieve in your personal, financial and professional life, starting with the next four weeks. Either in your journal or on a piece of paper, make a list of these goals.

★ Remember to choose goals that are within your control and measurable. Before deciding on a goal, ask yourself the intention behind it. Will it make you happier? More emotionally stable? More financially comfortable? Cast your mind back to the EEE method (see pages xxiv–xxv), and make these intentions as detailed as you can.

★ Also be honest with yourself and reflect on how continuing to drink in your current pattern may potentially block you from reaching these goals.

★ When you have made your list of goals for the next four weeks, if you like you can repeat this exercise by setting some goals for the next year.

★ If you haven't achieved all or any of your goals by the end of the month or the year, please don't give up on them; you can still do this, though it may take a bit more time and planning.

In a similar way to setting yourself SMART goals for what you'd like to achieve personally, professionally and financially, you can apply goal-setting to your relationship with alcohol. After all, we know that alcohol can impact people's lives in all of these areas, so it makes sense to think about setting ourselves goals for ourselves around our drinking too.

GOAL-SETTING AROUND YOUR SOBERISH JOURNEY

It's always useful to have a destination in mind during the course of any journey, so I'd like you to think now about what type of relationship with drinking you'd like to have. (It's OK, I'm not asking you to take an oath, sign your name in blood or commit to anything – this is about starting to find your own answers through the art of introspection.) Also, just to say that this isn't about replacing one set of labels with another. Instead, it might be helpful to think of the descriptions below as acting more like roadmaps that you can use to get yourself to where you think you'd like to be in relation to alcohol.

★ Mark the box or boxes that describe the kind of drinking habits that you aspire to have:

Type of drinker	Definition	✓
Soberish	You have taken your power back after alcohol misuse, but you may not be exclusively abstinent. Being soberish is about setting your intention, and working toward your own personalized goals with self-awareness and knowledge.	
Sober	You are abstinent from alcohol.	
Alcohol-free (AF)	You do not consume alcohol, but you may partake in other low-risk substances such as kava, THC, psilocybin or CBD.	
Sober curious	You are interested in the sober, alcohol-free or soberish lifestyle but you may not be ready to commit to full abstinence. You may have participated in a "Dry Month", cut back your alcohol intake or are exploring periods of sobriety for the health benefits of these.	
Low-risk drinker	You feel in control of your current drinking and have regular alcohol-free days. You stay within the recommended guidelines for moderate drinking. Overall, you can take it or leave it!	

Now that you have ticked your options, why not write down ways that you could apply the SMART goal technique and EEE method to them? (It might help to think in terms of achievable baby steps initially here.)

THE KEY STEPS IN A PLAN OF ACTION (POA)

If you're an athlete or at all familiar with sports then you know that a team doesn't just walk onto the field and "play ball"; they have a game plan. Can you imagine what would happen if professional athletes decided not to practise, warm up, become familiar with their plays or take the time to communicate with their teammates before the big game? Utter chaos – they'd essentially be walking into the game blind. This is how I view changing your relationship with alcohol without first creating a plan of action (POA), which we are going to be looking at in more detail in a moment. This plan will allow you to create awareness around your triggers, identify your responses and break the cycle of drinking. Knowing your drinking archetype is a great foundation for this POA, because it will give you an idea of where to start looking for your triggers. For example, if you tend to identify more as a stress drinker, you already know that stress and anxiety in general tend to lead you to drink. So your next step would be to figure out what exactly causes you stress.

In a nutshell, a POA is a detailed, written plan that you will create to help you foster new habits and behaviours so that alcohol no longer shows up in your life in a negative way. It can also be used to help you course-correct if a backslide occurs or you find yourself drinking more than you'd like to. This plan is an excellent resource to help support you and build a solid foundation on your new journey. It will consist of detailed resources, healthy coping mechanisms, people you can confide in and rely on, and future goal-setting options to help you stay focused.

When I created my first POA, it was early on in my journey. I realized quickly that unless I wanted to become a hermit and completely change my lifestyle, I would need to expose myself to things that made me uncomfortable – like going to bars, sober dating and hanging around other people who were drinking. When I first quit, I was 23 and still wanted to be a part of the Los Angeles nightlife and participate in what people my age were doing. It was difficult at first, but with the support of my friends and a strong POA I was able to navigate triggering scenarios and uncomfortable environments. After identifying which situations made me feel like drinking – like staying out until 2am when everyone else was plastered or working late nights at a bar – I shifted gears so I could keep my job and my friends, but also prioritize my current version of sobriety.

To take the pressure off "keeping up" with my drunk friends, I started to identify which gatherings and events felt appropriate for me to attend and which felt unnecessary. For example, I realized quickly that without alcohol or drugs I wasn't actually a fan of concerts or large crowds. The loud music and lack of space gave me anxiety and made whatever I was doing unenjoyable because I was massively overstimulated. This awareness was how I began to navigate my other triggers and eventually recognize the patterns of behaviour that caused them. With this new information in hand, I was able to happily decline invitations where I would be putting myself at risk of backsliding and kept myself open to gatherings that would feed my much smaller social butterfly without bleeding my Body Battery (we'll be looking at this concept in more detail on 231).

STEP ONE: IDENTIFYING OUR TRIGGERS

You've probably heard the word "trigger" before, as it gets thrown around pretty commonly these days. However, in order for us to be specific about our POA it's important to define exactly what a trigger is so that we can identify them. In psychology, a "trigger" is a stimulus that causes a painful memory to resurface. It can be any sensory reminder of a traumatic event: a sound, sight, smell, physical sensation, or even a time of day or season. For the sake of our POA, we are going to say that a trigger is any stimulus that leads us to drink. Identifying and becoming aware of your triggers can be difficult and uncomfortable at first, but it will strengthen your POA and set you up for success.

For me, although a handful of triggers have stayed the same over the years, my larger ones have changed over time. The process of "trigger changes" comes from getting older, becoming more mature (hopefully) and having healthier priorities. When I was 24, I was still going to clubs and enjoying late nights with my friends. Back then, I was triggered by loneliness, my untreated OCD and a fear of missing out on whatever my peers were doing. Now aged 30, I have learned how to enjoy my time alone and have a better relationship with myself, so I no longer fear being by myself or the thoughts that may come with this. In fact, more often than not when I see on their Instagram stories that my friends are out late, I experience JOMO (the joy of missing out), knowing I will be waking up hangover-free and without a face full of last night's makeup. Once I stopped drinking for a period of time, four years of abstinence to be specific, physiologically the medication I was prescribed for my OCD started working much better, which allowed me to regulate my emotions and use tools like therapy to become more stable and self-aware.

Everyone experiences triggers for different reasons, but there seems to be an overall consensus on what cues many of us to pick up the first drink in the early stages of our soberish journey. Knowing what these are can help you become more aware of your own triggers. Here are ten of the most common:

★ peer pressure
★ stress
★ social anxiety
★ sadness
★ loneliness
★ romanticizing others' drinking
★ happy hour
★ celebrations
★ hanging out in places you used to drink
★ getting into a fight with your partner

You may well be able to add a couple more of your own to the list.

STEP TWO: RECOGNIZING OUR RESPONSES

Identifying our unique triggers may seem difficult to do, but it becomes easier over time as we learn how to recognize what emotion we are feeling during the occurrence of a trigger. First, we need to understand that having a craving for alcohol or a strong desire to drink in a moment of discomfort is rarely about the alcohol itself. As a former triple-gin-and-tonic girl, I can say with confidence I never really craved the taste of a strong G&T because they taste like rubbing alcohol; what I was craving was an immediate relief from anxiety, social discomfort, sadness . . . the list goes on. For many of us, alcohol is a symptom and a temporary solution to something happening on

a deeper emotional level. We use alcohol as a way
to escape or avoid the way we feel – and it works,
for a moment. But what dulls today's edge sharpens
tomorrow and alcohol gives no free lunches. The
trade-off we make is rarely worth it and, more likely
than not, you've noticed by now that the negative
emotions you try to avoid are only exacerbated the
day after drinking.

So how do we begin to break the seemingly endless
cycle? As we've seen, we start by becoming more self-
aware. Rather than allowing our emotions to take the
driver's seat each time a trigger surfaces, we begin to
take note of when and where they occur. This is how
we begin to take our power back.

Below is a possible list of physical symptoms you
may feel when a trigger occurs; again, feel free to add
your own to these:

- ★ brain fog
- ★ chest tightness
- ★ rapid heart rate
- ★ nausea
- ★ shaking
- ★ heat flash
- ★ panic or fear

STEP THREE: ACTING ON OUR RESPONSES

Once we have started to notice and understand our
reactions in more detail, we can begin to make choices
about how to tackle these both in the moment and in
order to prevent them occurring more generally, using
the sorts of tools that we are going to be looking at in
more detail in Part Two of this book. With our newfound self-awareness, we can begin to frame different
types of response to use in specific situations that are

likely to arise for us, while keeping our longer-term soberish goals in mind.

STEP FOUR: RETRACING OUR STEPS

Now that we are becoming more aware of our emotional and physical responses, and perhaps have some emergency tools and coping strategies at our disposal that we can draw on, it's time to retrace our steps and calmly analyse what happened.

Let's create an example scenario. Say you have been working extremely hard on a new project. You present it to your manager and not only do they give you negative feedback but they decide it's also their job to give you unconstructive criticism – rude. Now, of course, you're upset – who wouldn't be? But it's the end of the work day and you're not going to put any more effort into the project tonight; you're upset and you just want to get out of there.

On the way home, you get a call from a friend to meet up at one of your favourite bars. You're not really in the mood but your friend pressures you into going, so you decide to stop by to say hi. You weren't planning on drinking, but you're still feeling attacked and angry from earlier, and you decide to have a few to unwind. You end up taking an Uber because you can't drive or cycle home, and now you are going to have to wake up early to go get your car or bike tomorrow before work. The day feels completely ruined and you go to bed upset, only to wake up early, unrested and still stewing in your new resentment for your boss. Not the best way to start a work day, or any day for that matter.

So what exactly happened here? Let's break it down:

★ You had no POA in place for a triggering situation such as being criticized by your boss.

★ You allowed your emotions to make decisions for you instead of following your instinct to go home.

★ Peer pressure got the better of you and ultimately led you to further poor decision-making.

This is what I like to call the snowball effect. It's very easy for us to fall into this trap if we don't have a POA in place or we are currently lacking the self-awareness to listen to our body instead of our emotions. Now, we may not be able to turn back time and change the situation, but we can better prepare ourselves for the next time something triggers us so that we are prepared. It's also important to note that not all of our triggers will make sense at first. Perhaps your boss is often critical and you've grown used to your boss's insensitivity, but on that particular day you had already been snapped at by your partner in the morning for forgetting to get tickets to this weekend's concert. Naturally you are already sensitive from the fight with your partner and your boss's feedback pushes you over the edge. Understanding the root cause of your negative stimulation can help you to address the real problem.

Triggers can also be deeper rooted than a simple spat with your partner. Perhaps you grew up in an environment where you were criticized regularly or told you weren't good enough by your parents? The way we view ourselves and how we react to situations can be formed in early adolescence, so while one person may not take their boss's criticism personally, you feel the sting of salt in an unhealed wound, bringing you back to a subconscious place of vulnerability and sadness. Here, in this place of unprocessed emotions, you find it easier to reach for a drink to escape how you feel than to take a deep breath and walk through the pain. Many of us feel this way and turn to distractions such as drinking, but the truth of the situation is that we will never truly heal until we address these unprocessed emotions, no matter how difficult they may be. The only way out is through.

STEP FIVE: REPEATING THE CYCLE OF AWARENESS

In the beginning of your journey, it will take some time before you are able to recognize all of your triggers, so be sure to practise self-compassion and patience. This process isn't linear by any means. Continue to take stock of your physical and emotional responses to situations and what emotions surface during a period of stimulation. Over time you will begin to recognize patterns in both your triggers and how you react to them.

Patterns can look like feeling social anxiety or "anticipation anxiety" before going out for the night, feeling overwhelmed every time you converse with a difficult person (such as an ex-partner, boss, or former friend), or always craving a drink once the clock hits 5pm. Being on the lookout for these patterns of emotions will help you develop more self-awareness and take intentional action with confidence.

Equipped with growing self-awareness, you can begin to put in place tactics and tools to help you deal with any challenging situations that may arise.

CREATING YOUR OWN PLAN OF ACTION

OK, so now you know what one looks like, it's time to draw up your own soberish Plan of Action. Let's go through this again one step at a time . . .

STEP ONE: IDENTIFY YOUR TRIGGERS

Remember that a trigger can be any stimulus that leads you to drink. With that definition in mind, I'd like you to write down in a journal, notebook or on your phone notes all of the triggers that you are currently aware of – all the people, places and things that lead you to drink. As you continue working with your POA, keep writing down any new triggers that come up or that you identify over time.

STEP TWO: RECOGNIZE YOUR RESPONSES

In order to recognize your responses, you must gain self-awareness. To do so, it's important to get curious about yourself and to have the courage to let down your emotional walls, rather than practise avoidance. From now on, when you notice yourself becoming overwhelmed by a powerful emotion, I want you to take stock of what you are experiencing and record this in your soberish journal, notepad or in the "notes" section of your phone, while asking yourself the following questions:

★ How am I feeling at the moment?
★ Do I feel angry, anxious, afraid or perhaps even jealous?

★ What about any physical signs: is my heart rate beginning to rise, am I breathing more heavily?

Remember that a response to a trigger can show up physiological symptoms such a tight chest, so use these reactions as clues to your triggers too, and create your own list of symptoms – both physical and emotional – that occur when you are experiencing a trigger or a craving. Feel free to keep coming back to this list and adding to it as you discover more.

STEP THREE: ACT ON YOUR RESPONSE

Think about how you responded to the triggers and the feelings that came up for you during these situations. What did you do? Could you have behaved differently? Was there anything that you could have said or done either during the situation, or more generally, that might have affected the outcome? What strategies or practices do you have at your disposal that could help you tackle future situations like this one? As mentioned, some of the tools described in Part Two can be very helpful to implement at this stage of your POA.

STEP FOUR: RETRACE YOUR STEPS

Now that you are becoming more aware of your responses and your choices around them, begin to revisit the different situations in which you have been triggered that led you to drink or to almost drink. Here are some questions to ask yourself:

★ What was I doing directly before I became overstimulated?

★ Was there a specific moment in which I felt the negative emotion come up, or was it a gradual build-up of smaller triggers?

★ Was I talking to someone specific before or when I felt the desire to drink?

Write down your answers and reflect on this going forward.

STEP FIVE: REPEAT THE CYCLE OF AWARENESS

Continue to take stock of your physical and emotional responses to situations and notice what emotions surface during a period of stimulation. Over time you will begin to recognize patterns in both your triggers and how you react to them, and you will also start to have an array of tools in place to help you deal with these.

To give you a sense of what a Plan of Action could look like, here is a very simplified example using a specific scenario – the possibility of bumping into an ex at an important social event:

1. You know that you are still very triggered by your ex, who broke your heart. To make matters worse, you have been invited to attend the wedding of close mutual friends, and your ex will be there too, making this potentially a very emotionally charged event for you.

2. You recognize that you still feel incredibly hurt by this past relationship and you are anxious that you won't be able to keep your emotions under control when you see your ex at the wedding. To make

things worse, even though you care deeply about your friends who are getting married, you can't help feeling jealous that they are about to enjoy the sort of happy-ever-after that you never got to experience with your ex.

③ Nonattendance of events like this one is not an option for you, but you know you can draw on the tools of sleep and mindfulness (see Part Two) to help you rest and soothe your anxiety beforehand. And if you do start to panic at the event, you can quickly calm yourself down using box breathing (see page 163).

④ At the wedding, you tune in to how you feel at each stage. Is it as bad as you thought it would be, and how do you handle any emotions that came up for you?

⑤ Finally, you can ask yourself whether it would be helpful to do anything differently next time there is a social event at which your ex will be present. Were those tools useful, for example, or could you use any other tools to help you face your ex next time without wanting to drown your sorrows in the nearest bar?

Take your time when creating your own POA; this isn't a quick fix and you're done, but a process that you can keep revisiting and refining as much as you like during the course of your soberish journey. The better prepared and equipped you are to recognize your responses and deal with potential situations and setbacks, the more rewarding your journey is likely to be.

YOU'RE ALL SET . . .

By now, you hopefully have a much better understanding of how the brain can work for us as well as against us when it comes to shaping our attitudes, impulses and behaviours generally around alcohol. You are likely a lot more aware of your own drinking patterns and your triggers too, and generally have a clearer understanding of your personal relationship with alcohol. As we've seen, self-awareness really is key, even when this can take us to some uncomfortable places.

In light of what you've discovered so far, you may have already set yourself some SMART goals and intentions and drafted the beginnings of your own soberish Plan of Action around them. (If you haven't got round to this yet, there's still time.) All in all, you're developing a clearer idea of what a soberish lifestyle could look like for you, so now you need the means to make this lifestyle a reality. In Part Two, we are going to put together a toolkit to help you achieve exactly that.

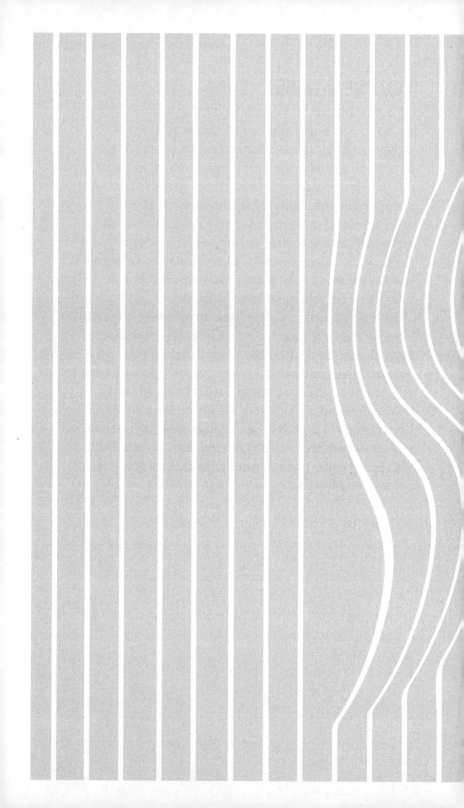

Creating Your Soberish Toolkit

CREATING YOUR SOBERISH TOOLKIT

As you pursue a soberish way of living, it's critical you continue to reinforce the healthy outlets you are creating. You want the old neural pathways that cue you to drink to whither, while you nourish new pathways that lead you to healthier habits. This is done through repetition and finding activities to add to your soberish toolkit that you can easily include in your POA and which will bring you happiness and stability. Tools can come in all shapes and sizes; once you get the hang of this, you may find many others that reflect your own interests and talents. Everyone's toolkit will look different, and that's OK – it's a reminder that we are all individuals who drink for different reasons and come from a wide range of environmental circumstances. We don't all drink the same way, so why would our toolkit look the same?

What I've found most important about having a toolkit is that it's heavily reliant on the self. If you have tools that are easily accessible and are based within your own sphere of control, you hold the power to navigate any situation in your favour. This is why I have chosen some evidence-based and self-controlled tools from my own toolkit to share with you. These range from supportive practices such as eating well and getting a good night's sleep, to somatic intuition and cold therapy.

While you don't have to read the chapters in Part Two in any particular order, and are free to dip into them in whichever way seems most helpful to you, you will discover that they do build upon each other, from creating a solid base through tools such as diet and sleep, to physical activities like intuitive movement, to those that promote good mental health, such as mindfulness and journaling. The reason for this is that having a solid bedrock of supportive practices in place will help you to get the most out of other tools too. As an example, I don't know if you've ever tried meditating when you are tired and hungry? If you have, you'll probably remember that you nearly dozed off or ended up distracted by your growling stomach.

Feeling a craving or trigger emotion coming on? Using the self-awareness afforded by your POA and drawing upon the tools you have available to you that do not involve alcohol will help you to redirect your energy into something positive that will ultimately benefit you in the short and long term. All of these tools have scientifically proven benefits and each of them has continued to serve me well over the years. It's my sincere hope and belief that you are going to find them just as helpful as I have on your own soberish journey.

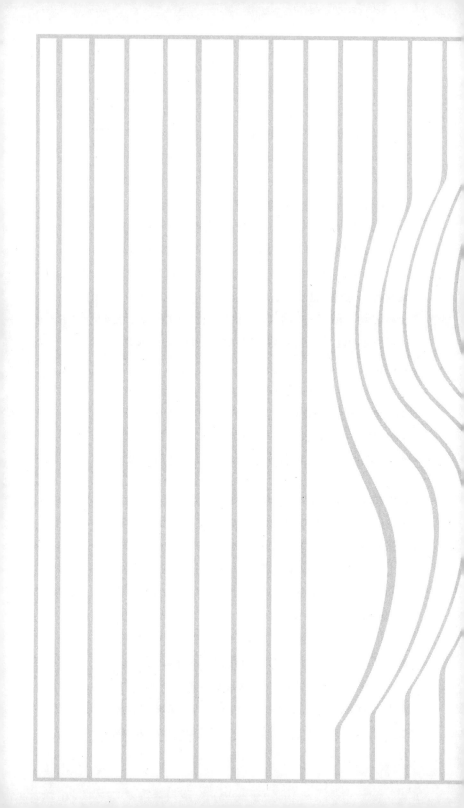

CHAPTER 5

Eat Well: Nourish Your Body's Second Brain

Have you ever wondered if the food you're consuming is affecting your ability to change your relationship with alcohol? The simple answer is *yes*. Poor diet and nutrient deficiencies can lead to cravings and alcohol misuse, as well as play an ongoing role in the formation of alcohol use disorder (AUD). Nutrient deficiencies and insufficient production of amino acids (molecules in your body that form protein) can lead to imbalances in your body, leaving you at higher risk of alcohol misuse and potentially undoing any progress you've made in taking control over your relationship with drinking.

Why is this? Because your gut works like your body's "second brain", the imbalances in your microbiome turn into imbalances in your hormones, which then lead to emotional and mental health irregularities. As we've discussed, deficiency or impairment of our neurochemicals such as dopamine or GABA can be caused by alcohol misuse – but not just from damage caused by alcohol to the brain. What most people don't know is that these neurotransmitters aren't just a product of our brain: some of them or their precursors are also synthesized in the gut. This means that if the gut is in a state of dysregulation from nutritional deficiencies, it will not allow for the formation or proper functioning of some of these neurotransmitters. The worse these deficiencies become over time, the more likely a person is to continue drinking and the harder it is for them to stop.

When you consider the whole body and the impact that drinking has on the gut, you begin to realize the power alcohol has over your entire system. Alcohol can have detrimental effects on all of your internal processes – and this includes the gut microbiome, the trillions of bacteria in your intestines that aid digestion and which help support the body's immune system. Both good and potentially harmful bacteria exist inside of us at all times and the gut microbiome is responsible for helping to keep our bodies in balance.

When we consume alcohol, especially large amounts and in high concentrations, we can overwhelm our gastrointestinal tract. This kills off the good bacteria, leading to bacterial overgrowth which can cause heartburn, bile acid build-up, sour stomach, inflammation of the gut and dysbiosis (a microbial imbalance that can lead to disease).[1] Even more alarming, this good bacteria plays a crucial role in influencing your neural, immune and endocrine pathways,[2] which means that harming it can impact your mental health negatively. Supported by the right foods and supplementation, you stand a much better chance of repairing your gut microbe, improving your overall health and preventing future backslides when it comes to sustaining a new relationship with alcohol.

IMPROVING YOUR DIET

There are a few specific areas of your diet you can focus on in the beginning of your journey that will help you repair and replenish your nutrient deficiencies. The first area you want to focus on is *fibre*. "Consuming fibre will help you to rebalance your gut bacteria that has been dysregulated by alcohol consumption," nutritionist Dr Brooke Scheller, creator of Functional Sobriety, tells me when I speak to her over Zoom, adding, "Fibre is food for your gut microbes, which will assist in replenishing your digestive system with good bacteria."[3] The American Heart Association Eating Plan suggests that we eat 25 to 30 grammes of fibre from foods – not supplements – per day.[4] We can source our daily intake of fibre from vegetables, beans, berries, nuts and whole grains.

NUTRIENT-DENSE FOODS

Because alcohol misuse can cause nutrient depletion, it's also important to focus on adding foods to your diet that are nutrient-dense, meaning they have high vitamin and mineral content in relation to their weight. To re-establish a healthy diet, eat sources of lean proteins such as fish or lentils, fruits, vegetables, beans, whole grains and sources of healthy fats like nuts and seeds. Here are some suggestions to get you started:

Fruits and vegetables

The powerhouses of nutrient-dense foods, fruits and veggies are packed with vitamins, minerals, fibre, phytochemicals and antioxidants – all important nutrients that may be depleted from alcohol misuse. Some of my personal favourites are spinach, broccoli, kale, carrots, Brussels sprouts (OK, not everybody's favourite!), sweet potatoes, berries, bananas and avocados.

Lean proteins

Protein is an important nutrient for our muscles, brain and skin, and can help you fight off the kind of sugar cravings that can occur when we start drinking less. This is because alcohol is converted to sugar in the body, which leads to spikes in our blood sugar levels, and when we cut back on booze, our body can feel deprived. On top of this, sugar affects the brain's pleasure centre much like alcohol does, and can give us a similar buzz.[5] (See page 109, where nutritionist Kiola Raines goes into this in more detail.) Protein will help stabilize your blood sugar levels and keep you feeling full for longer, which can offset those "sweet tooth" impulses. Lean meat cuts like skinless chicken or turkey, and beans, eggs, tofu and seafood are excellent sources of B vitamins, iron and zinc.

Research has shown that these particular nutrients tend to be deficient in those people who struggle with alcohol use disorders.[6]

Whole grains

Naturally high in fibre, whole grains can help you to maintain a healthy gut microbiome and also keep you feeling satiated. Whole grains are a great resource for other important nutrients as well, such as B vitamins, iron, folate, selenium, potassium and magnesium.[7] I'm a fan of oatmeal, brown rice and plain popcorn to get my fill of grains.

Nuts

Easily my favourite snack foods, nuts! Nuts are a great source of fibre, healthy fats and plant protein. Nuts such as almonds, pistachios, peanuts and pecans are also a great source for nutrients, like vitamins and minerals – not to mention they are oh-so tasty!

Beans

Beans, beans, the magical fruit! For all my plant-based friends, beans or legumes are a good source of plant-protein as well as fibre. Beans are great because they can be incorporated into so many different kinds of dishes like tacos, soups, stews and salads. They can also be found in dips like hummus and salsa.

"Different types of foods can provide benefits to the different systems in your body that have been negatively impacted by alcohol, like your stomach, liver and heart," explains Dr Scheller. "Consuming these nutrient-dense foods, and herbs like turmeric and ginger, will help with your body's natural detoxification processes as well." Yes, you really can eat your way to better health!

DIETARY SUPPLEMENTATION

Alcohol disrupts the way we eat in a variety of ways, so it's important to keep in mind that if you are a habitual heavy drinker, or prone to the occasional binge, you more than likely have nutritional deficiencies due to your alcohol consumption. "Alcohol affects your appetite, your food choices, many acute and chronic disease states, and the ability for your gut lining to effectively absorb nutrients," my friend Jeff Simone tells me in our email exchange.[8] Jeff is a doctor of pharmacy and certified advanced dietary supplement adviser, and he explains, "Heavy drinking also causes a direct loss of certain micronutrients that are necessary for a healthy diet. Vitamins B1, B2, B5, and Zinc, for example." Even if you're not experiencing visible signs or symptoms, these nutritional deficiencies can lead to feelings of distress or discomfort at the beginning of your soberish journey, whatever your starting point or goals in relation to drinking.

The long-term plan to get ourselves to a place of balance has to include looking at our diet too, so that we can reverse any damage caused by malnutrition or blood-sugar abnormalities. As part of this, dietary supplementation should strongly be considered at the beginning to help kick-start the process. "When combined with sensible nutrition, supplementation can help repair the damaged cells, moderate the impact of stress and illness, and reduce infection risk," explains Dr Simone. "The goal of any combination of vitamins, minerals, amino acids, and other nutrients is three-fold: to help the body 'cleanse' from the physical effects of alcohol, eliminate cravings, and significantly reduce potential withdrawal symptoms."

Recommended supplements include a range of vitamins and amino acids. While these occur naturally in many foods, supplements can be very helpful sources in times of need. However, like most things in life, taking too much or for too long can have harmful side effects, so always read the packaging and, whenever possible, consult a healthcare professional before making significant changes to your diet, such as taking certain types of supplement.[9]

Vitamins and minerals

Vitamins and minerals are organic compounds that are essential for the proper functioning of the body, as they are needed for the healthy growth, development and function of cells. The following are all readily available as supplements:

★ **Multivitamin or multimineral:** A good-quality multivitamin or multimineral is the keystone of a basic supplement regimen for detoxing the body of alcohol and rebalancing the system. Standard multivitamins and multiminerals will provide the recommended daily allowance (RDA) for most vitamins and minerals, many of which can become depleted in a person's body over the course of many years of heavy alcohol consumption.

★ **B-vitamin complex:** Because they have similar biochemical structures, the B-vitamins often get grouped together and can be acquired as a "complex" that includes most, if not all, of them. Many individuals with AUD have deficiencies in several specific B-vitamins, which is why it is recommended that they take a B-complex rather than individual vitamins.

★ **Vitamin C:** This water-soluble vitamin acts as an antioxidant. It protects the body from free radicals (unstable molecules that can cause damage to other molecules), assists in the metabolism of the amino acid tryptophan (which is the precursor to feel-good serotonin), stimulates adrenal activity, and performs a range of other critical functions. "You can safely take 1 to 3g of Vitamin C daily in divided doses. If you experience diarrhoea or loose stools, the dose should be lowered," explains Dr Jeff Simone.

★ **Magnesium:** A deficiency of magnesium can disrupt an individual's ability to sleep and make us feel more depressed, moody and irritable. This is why magnesium consumption can help reduce uncomfortable symptoms like these, which may be experienced after quitting alcohol or significantly cutting back. Dr Simone tells me that, "There are many salt forms of magnesium on the market, but I recommend magnesium glycinate or magnesium threonate. These forms are easier on the stomach and can typically improve sleep patterns relatively quickly." Although magnesium supplements can be taken earlier in the day, he typically recommends they should be taken one hour before bed for best effect.

★ **Omega-3:** These essential fatty acids act as anti-inflammatory agents throughout the brain and body and are critical for reducing inflammation and preventing disease. Fatty acids in the brain also increase the production of serotonin, thereby reducing depressive symptoms. "A 1,500 mg omega-3 fish or krill oil supplement is an effective way to obtain this nutrient if you are not eating two to three servings a week of fatty fish – e.g. salmon, tuna, anchovies, mackerel, herring, etc.," explains Dr Simone.

Amino acids

Amino acids are the building blocks of proteins. They're also considered the principal source of the neurotransmitters in the brain such as serotonin, dopamine, GABA, norepinephrine and epinephrine. If your diet is well balanced, you will receive most of the nutrients you need through the food you consume. However, as mentioned earlier, most of us who may overconsume alcohol do not typically have well-balanced diets. So, more than likely, we will be deficient in amino acids. "Many researchers and clinicians, as well as many peer-reviewed research articles, agree that amino acid therapy can speed up the restoration of normal brain function in those with AUD," explains Dr Simone, "thereby reducing cravings, lessening symptoms of depression, boosting energy, and reducing anxiety."

Because there are a limited number of transporters for amino acids in our gut, it is recommended that they be taken on an empty stomach (at least 30 mins before or two hours after meals) so the protein from your food does not reduce the absorption of the amino acid supplements by competing for transport through the small intestine.

The following supplements are generally considered safe, but as mentioned earlier, please do seek the advice of a trained healthcare professional who is familiar with the nuances and details of your lifestyle and your medical and psychological history before adding these to your diet. I would also caution strongly against beginning to take amino acid supplements while taking prescription psychotropic medications.

* **Glutamine:** This is a precursor to GABA (a neurotransmitter that improves memory, helps the body relax, and reduces cravings for alcohol). Dr Simone says, "I have observed

many individuals quench a sudden urge to drink alcohol by opening a 500mg glutamine capsule and dissolving the contents under the tongue (sublingual absorption is much quicker than oral absorption through the GI tract)."

★ **Tyrosine:** An essential amino acid that is needed for the formation of the specific neurotransmitters (i.e. dopamine, epinephrine, norepinephrine). It also helps form important brain chemicals that affect mood and sleep. Tyrosine can help us cope with the physical stress of detoxification. However, it's important to note that other vitamins and minerals like B-vitamins, vitamin C and copper, etc., are needed for proper tyrosine metabolism.

★ **5-HTP:** 5-Hydroxytryptophan (5-HTP) is a precursor to serotonin. As serotonin plays a key role in regulating our sleep and our moods, I'd strongly suggest providing your body with this important precursor to help offset the common complaints of sleeplessness and low mood when first cutting down or quitting drinking. To convert 5-HTP to serotonin, your body must also be getting adequate amounts of magnesium and several B-vitamins.

★ **Methionine:** An essential amino acid that supports memory, prevents fatigue and has been shown to provide relief for depressive symptoms.

★ **L-theanine:** An amino acid that is unique in its ability to produce almost immediate relaxation. L-theanine is found naturally in green tea, which can help to balance caffeine's jitteriness effects. It can relieve anxiety, low mood and insomnia. It works by acting on the brain's

GABA/glutamate system by tipping the scales in the direction of relaxation versus excitability. Jeff Simone says, "Because the effects of post-acute withdrawal syndrome (PAWS) can be so pronounced and long-standing in heavier drinkers, I typically recommend supplementation with L-theanine for several months or until symptoms fully resolve."

As you can see, supplements can be useful to have in your toolkit. However, for readers based in the USA, it should be noted that because the FDA does not have the authority to approve dietary supplements for safety and effectiveness, and nor do they approve a product's labelling before being sold to the public, it is the consumer's responsibility to ensure the products are of high quality. When considering a dietary supplement, look for those with the NSF, NPA or USP seal: this means the product meets or exceeds Good Manufacturing Practices (GMP) standards for quality. "Products that have opted not to pursue these seals of approval might well be avoided," says Dr Simone. "It is also recommended to take these nutrients in capsule form if possible, as this delivery mechanism is typically much more readily broken down and absorbed compared to hard-pressed tablets." In the UK, there is no requirement to register food supplements. As long as they comply with the laws specific to food supplements and all other applicable food law, they are permitted for sale. It is the responsibility of the manufacturer, importer or retailer to ensure that they comply with the law – but there can be no guarantees that products sourced on the internet will do this. Wherever you live in the world, it's worth doing some proper research into the products that are available and the government guidelines and recommendations for these. The soberish journey is all about self-care, which means finding the time and resources to start looking after yourself properly.

TALKING WITH A NUTRITION EXPERT

Kiola Raines is a self-confessed wellness geek, Precision Nutrition certified coach and a National Academy of Sports Medicine certified trainer. She generously took some time out of her busy schedule to chat to me about the role that nutrition can play in our soberish journey. As someone who has transformed her own relationship with alcohol, she has some great advice on getting started on changing your diet and then sustaining those changes. My questions are in italic, with her answers below.

How can someone get started creating a healthier nutrition plan?
Increasing health starts with increasing the nutrient density of our meals and snacks. So far, your readers have learned about the important macro- and micronutrients that can benefit the soberish journey, and the next step is implementation. Once you have determined your unique nutritional needs, start by adding in one key macro- or micronutrient at a time. Rather than giving your current diet an overhaul, start with a slower, more sustainable approach. Pick the nutrient you want to implement first and start adding it into your meals and snacks. For example, if your nutrient focus is protein, start including protein portions in each of your meals and snacks. You will know exactly how much protein to add, based on your unique nutritional needs. Once you are meeting your

protein needs consistently, choose another key nutrient and begin adding it into your daily menu.

It's likely the reader will run into sugar cravings, so how should they deal with them in a healthy way?
First, I think it's important for folks to know why you are experiencing the sugar cravings in the first place. As a person in recovery myself, I wish I had an understanding of the sugar cravings early on, so let's start with why they're happening. It comes down to dopamine and our reward system. Substance use interferes with our brain's communication/chemical messages, and its ability to reward us for positive behaviours. With continued use or abuse, the body begins to operate and expect unnatural levels of dopamine, for a negative behaviour. When you remove the dopamine source, this cycle is interrupted, but your brain knows there are alternate ways to keep the cycle going, and on come the sugar cravings.

So let's talk about dealing with and learning from the cravings. It all comes down to nutrient density and having a plan. Start by stocking up on all of your favourite fruits; this is a nutrient-dense way to move through the craving. Along with a dose of sweet, you're also getting vitamins, minerals and fibre. If you pair your fruit with a handful of nuts, the fat plus protein will help balance blood sugar after enjoying a sweet treat. For the times when fruit just won't do the job, and if you find yourself eating candy, cookies, ice cream and the like, pairing those sweets with a protein or fat is still key. My go-to is a scoop of chocolate protein powder and ice cold water in a shaker; it's easyand quick to make and pairs perfectly with chocolate chip cookies!

Why is regulating your blood sugar so important?
And how can the reader learn to use food and
supplementation to regulate their system?
When ideal glucose levels in blood are maintained, our
brain and body can operate at optimal levels. If blood
sugar levels dip low or spike high, this disrupts the
body's communication, which can lead to cravings. Two
simple ways to avoid this are eating often and eating
nutrient-dense, balanced meals. A general rule of thumb
is to have some nutrients within an hour of waking,
and to continue eating every three hours, to keep a
steady balance of glucose in the blood. I suggested
pairing sweets with fat or protein to avoid the glucose
spike that sweets can cause to our system. Balance all
of your meals and snacks by including a serving of
protein and fat along with carbohydrates. If you
want to experience a balanced mood, clear thinking
and steady energy, plus the ultimate bonus of fewer
cravings, learn to balance your blood sugar.

How would you recommend integrating a sustainable
nutrition programme to people in the beginning of
their soberish journey?
The key to a sustainable nutrition programme is
creating a plan that you enjoy and can ultimately
commit to for years to come. When it comes to
implementing this type of nutrition in the beginning
of a soberish journey, I suggest starting slowly, building
effective nutrition habits one at a time. For many, this
is not the ideal time for a complete nutrition overhaul.
If you're considering changing the way you're eating,
get with a certified professional to determine your
unique nutritional needs. Some folks may benefit
from lab-testing for nutrient and neurotransmitter
deficiencies, or impaired organ function as a result

of substance use. Once you have a clear picture of your body's specific needs, work alongside a certified professional as you learn to create your own enjoyable, sustainable programme, implementing one effective nutrition habit at a time.

What are the top three "myths" people believe about food?

1. Food is fuel, like gasoline for a car. Food is actually information, similar to data, for a computer. The food we eat contains the data our bodies need in order to send the messages to our organs which allow our bodies to function.

2. You can't eat your ethnic or cultural foods and achieve health. Nutrient density is the focus of an effective nutrition plan, and this can be achieved with foods from all cultures and ethnicities.

3. Don't eat anything you can't pronounce. The truth is every single plant, fruit, grain – literally every food item – has a biochemical makeup that some folks may not be able to pronounce. The aroma of food has a biochemical makeup, the flavour of food and colour of food as well. This is one of the most harmful myths floating around, because it creates fear around food.

EAT YOURSELF WELL

Whatever your attitude to eating, by adjusting your diet it may become easier each day to ward off the sort of cravings that usually have you reaching for the bottle.

★ Keep a food diary for a week. This isn't about calorie counting, but about becoming more aware of what you eat on a day-to-day basis. Does your diet look balanced, with a variety of vegetables and fruit?

★ When you eat, take an honest look at your plate: what are you really feeding yourself? Is it likely to help you deal with your cravings or to tip your blood-sugar levels into freefall?

★ Actively find ways to include more nutrient-dense foods in your diet such as vegetables and nuts. Step by step, swap out food that is heavy in saturated fat, sugar and salt for healthier options.

★ Can you swap out booze and sodas for glasses of water and unsweetened fruit juice?[10]

★ Consider taking a supplement or two, especially in the early stages of your soberish journey – but always read the packaging carefully and seek advice from healthcare professionals before making any major changes to your diet.

★ Make a note of which nutrient-dense foods make you feel physically and mentally stronger, so that you can include them more often in your diet.

FOOD FOR THOUGHT

The soberish journey is all about finding opportunities to enjoy more of the good things in life – and for many of us that includes food. If your drinking habits tend toward those of the social or sensory drinker, including food in your toolkit could be especially rewarding, giving you the opportunity to seek out and socialize with likeminded people and/or explore how to feed yourself, body and soul, in ways that will enable you to stave off sugar and booze cravings and take back control of your narrative when it comes to alcohol. For those whose drinking behaviours veer more toward drunkorexia, food will likely be an extremely challenging topic in its own right, so please seek any professional support you may need in this area.

Whatever your relationship with eating, the great news is that you can literally eat your way to optimum health through a balanced diet that includes plenty of nutrient-dense foods. These contain the fibre, vitamins, minerals and things like amino acids that are needed for our physical and mental wellbeing. Even if food doesn't usually feature high on your list of priorities, the next time you are tempted to reach for the cookie jar, maybe snack on an apple or a handful of almonds instead. If you don't usually spend much time in the kitchen, perhaps make cooking yourself nutritional meals part of your POA for the week? However, before changing your diet completely, do consult a healthcare professional such as your doctor or a nutritionist who can offer you individually tailored guidance.

As well as helping you to improve your mental and physical wellbeing, and creating a solid footing that will enable you to reshape your relationship with alcohol, eating well is a simple yet natural way to be kind to yourself, as is the next tool in our kit: sleep.

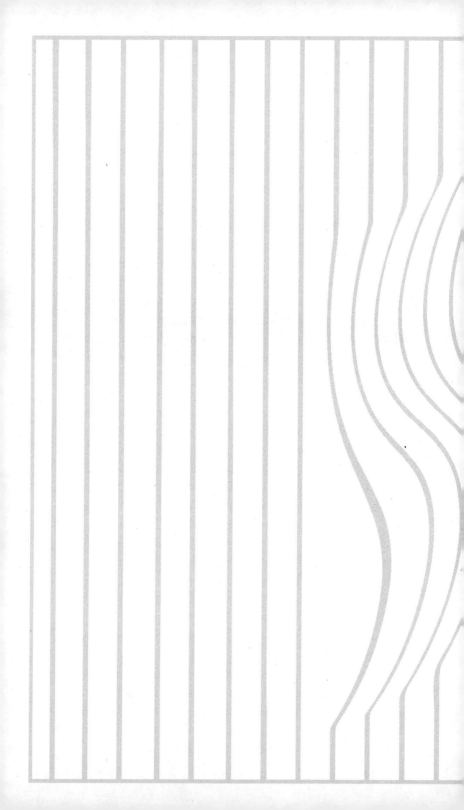

CHAPTER 6

Sleep On It: The Healing Power of Rest

As humans, we spend on average a third of our life sleeping – that's a good chunk. Sleep is important for so many aspects of whole-body healing, such as increasing our blood flow, which helps muscles recover and reduces inflammation in the body. This in turn helps us relieve stress and produce the hormones we need to repair and form new cells.[1] While we all know sleep is important, most of us probably don't realize just how much proper sleep deeply impacts our daily functions, overall wellbeing and mental health, which is why it really is important to get a good night's sleep.

Sleep is considered an essential bodily function: without enough of it, your brain can have a hard time performing basic functions and a lack of sleep increases your risk of disease. It becomes difficult to make informed choices, such as how to cope in stressful situations that might make you feel like drinking. You may even drink because you think it helps you to relax, when it can actually affect the quality of rest that you get. While you may still be getting seven to nine hours of sleep when you drink, the major issue is the impact alcohol can have on your quality of sleep. Poor sleep can result in a cycle of mental health deterioration, mood swings and a lack of energy.

I genuinely never realized how much my sleep quality was impacted by alcohol until I stopped drinking. I spent from age 16 to 23 drinking heavily almost every night without a single thought of the damage I was doing to my bodily functions. Like many of us, I was under the impression that alcohol helped me fall asleep, when in reality I was really just passing out most nights. Eventually, I felt like I needed a glass or two to relax my mind enough to drift off, but even though I seemed to be out like a light, what I mistaking for deep sleep was really just unconsciousness.

One of the first things to know if you want to sleep better is the role alcohol plays in your sleep. While many people assume alcohol helps them sleep better, it actually does quite the opposite. During the night, when your liver enzymes metabolize the alcohol you've consumed that day, you actually experience a decrease in the quality of sleep and are more likely to have sleep disruptions. You may also notice more fatigue the day after you drink because of this. Alcohol decreases the number of REM (Rapid Eye Movement) cycles that you go through while you sleep, so even if you sleep the same number of hours you normally would, you miss out on the deep, restorative sleep you need to recover and regenerate.[2]

PRACTISING PROPER SLEEP HYGIENE

Sleep hygiene is a term used to describe good sleeping habits. It can be practised through establishing a consistent environment and daily routine,[3] which is the easiest way to set yourself up for deeper, more restful sleep.

• •

DO YOU PRACTISE GOOD SLEEP HYGIENE?

Here is a quick quiz to find out whether you practise good sleep hygiene. Check any of the points that apply to you in the following list:

☐ You have a hard time falling asleep.
☐ You experience frequent sleep disturbances.
☐ You suffer from daytime sleepiness/fatigue.

☐ You nap often.

☐ You go to bed at different types and have no
set sleep/wake-up times or routine.

These are all signs of poor sleep hygiene, and the more
points you scored, the likelier it is that you need to
address your bedtime habits. There are many causes
of poor sleep hygiene. Check any that apply to you:

☐ Watching TV or being on your phone before bed.

☐ A bedroom that has temperature extremes.

☐ Taking too many naps or napping for too long
during the day.

☐ Spending time in bed doing things other than
sleeping like watching TV, scrolling through
your phone, eating.

☐ Having irregular bedtimes and getting up at
different times in the morning.

☐ Having a non-active lifestyle.

☐ Exercising right before bedtime.

☐ Having a caffeine or alcohol intake.

If none of these apply to you, congratulations! But if
you have checked anything on the list, it's likely you
have an issue with sleep hygiene. So let's fix that.

• •

SET YOURSELF UP FOR SUCCESSFUL SLEEP

Cutting back or ditching alcohol can be a great first
step in helping you sleep significantly better. While
the first few weeks will probably feel a little wonky,

be aware that your body is getting used to relearning how to regulate on its own. If your sleep is suffering, hang tight, as here are a few tips and tricks you can use to help get a better night's rest.

Upgrade your environment

Where you sleep is a foundational piece of proper sleep hygiene. At bedtime, keep your lights dim or off, and don't use your screens once you get into bed.[4] Light of any kind but especially blue light can hinder the production of melatonin, the sleep hormone your body naturally produces.[5] You can also talk to your doctor about melatonin supplementation to tide you over. The secret to melatonin is to take it when the sun goes down, not right before bed. It usually takes a couple of hours to start working.[6] Make sure your bedroom is quiet, comfortable and a relaxing place to be.

Find the perfect bedroom temperature

The best bedroom temperature for sleep is approximately 18°C (65°F). If your room is too hot, this can cause discomfort and restlessness. In fact, a National Sleep Foundation poll found that a cool room temperature was one of the most important factors in getting a good night's sleep, with as many as four out of five respondents saying this was important to them.[7] If you don't have air conditioning, there are a few ways you can keep your room cool: keep the blinds closed during the day, keep the windows open for ventilation, and purchase cooling or breathable sheets. You can also take a hot bath a couple of hours before bed to encourage a natural cool-down effect.[8]

Try using aromatherapy

Aromatherapy has been used as a form of healing therapy since ancient times. Modern research suggests that essential oils can create a bedroom environment that is more conducive to falling and staying asleep.[9] Expose your nose to pleasant smells such as lavender, rose and jasmine, which are associated with a positive mood, calmness and relaxation. Lavender has been linked with improved sleep in multiple sleep research studies as it helps lower the heart rate and blood pressure, as well as elevate mood. In a study of people exposed to lavender before bedtime, their levels of deep sleep increased, leading to them feeling more refreshed in the morning.[10]

Create a bedtime routine – and stick to it!

Your daytime routine affects your circadian rhythm, your body's internal clock that helps to carry out essential functions and processes, the most important of which is controlling the sleep–wake cycle and the homeostatic regulation of sleep. The longer we are awake, the more the pressure for sleep builds up in our body.[11] Sleep–wake homeostasis also impacts how alert or tired we feel during the day. To keep a balanced sleep–wake cycle it is important to have consistent daily habits. If you don't follow a routine, try to create one by going to bed at the same time each night and getting up at the same in the morning, even at the weekend.

Get your daily intake of vitamin D

Sunlight is one of the key drivers of the circadian rhythm, which can encourage quality sleep. So go outside for a brisk walk each day, even if it's cloudy.

Practice intuitive movement

Regular movement during the day can make it easier to sleep at night and also delivers a host of other health benefits, many of which we will be talking about in chapter 7. However, make sure not to work out too close to bedtime, as the endorphins may keep you awake.

Limit your intake of nicotine and caffeine!

Nicotine, like caffeine, stimulates the body in ways that disrupt sleep and cause a host of other issues like cancer and lung disease. Caffeine can keep you wired even when you want to rest, so try to avoid it after 3pm.[12]

Don't eat too late

Eating dinner late, especially if it's a large meal, can mean you're still digesting when it's time for bed, which goes against your body's circadian rhythm. Don't go to bed hungry, but any food or snacks before bed should be on the lighter side, such as a banana with almond butter, crackers and cheese, trail mix or a plain yogurt.

NIGHT, NIGHT!

Imagine how great you are going to feel after a good night's sleep. Sleep is such an important part of our wellbeing, it's worth paying it some serious attention and taking whatever steps you can to improve your sleep hygiene. If your drinking habits resemble those of the stress drinker or the self-medicating drinker, good-quality sleep could be an essential part of your soberish toolkit, enabling you to think more clearly and to feel more in charge of your waking life, reducing the impulse to use alcohol as a shortcut to relaxation at the end of the day or as a distraction from your problems.

If you find that thoughts are whirring round in your head, maybe keep a journal to hand where you can jot them down quickly, to deal with during the daytime. Sleep is essential to every process in the body, and you deserve to enjoy your rest as much as you do your waking hours. Talking of which, it's time now to find your flow, through intuitive movement . . .

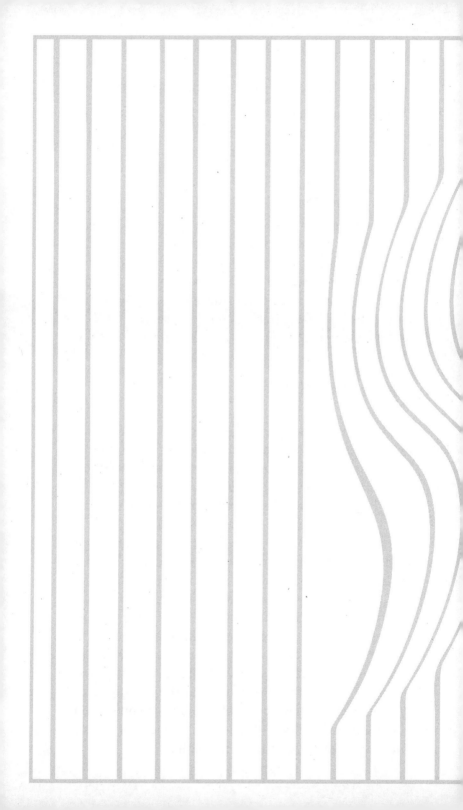

CHAPTER 7

Find Your Flow: Intuitive Movement

It's safe to assume that you've heard exercise plays an important role in your overall health. Over the last ten years there's been a huge fitness movement in the Western world, encouraging people to get in the gym or become active in other ways. Popular fitness boutiques and workout equipment for the home have sprouted up like weeds. While breaking a sweat continues to play an integral role in my own soberish journey, I've found that intuitive movement is even more purposeful when it comes to maintaining my overall wellbeing.

According to Lindsay Dalton, a registered yoga teacher and trauma-informed breathwork facilitator, the difference between intuitive movement and general movement is the intention behind it. "Intuitive movement is about letting go of an outcome, like losing weight or any expectation of how you think you should feel, and shifting to what your body needs in that moment. It will look different every day, reflecting the natural ebb and flow of life," she explains to me when we meet. "Practising this state of mind increases your 'felt sense' over time. This is our ability to step out of the mind and feel, notice and name sensations that we are experiencing in our body, which allows us to show up with intention and authenticity." Rather than focusing on sticking to a rigid workout routine, keep asking yourself questions like, "What are my energy levels today?" and "What is my intention behind today's exercise?"

Before I started practising intuitive movement, I had a nasty habit of over-exercising. After taking alcohol out of the picture as a stress-reduction tool, I jumped head first into fitness; some would call this a *transfer addiction*. And I know they say you can't have too much of a good thing, but that isn't exactly true.

For someone like me, who also suffers from disordered eating and a negative body image, over-exercising can be a slippery slope back into a full-blown eating disorder (ED). And given that research shows that the comorbidity rate of substance abuse and eating disorders is up to 27 per cent,[1] I am willing to bet many people reading this book are at risk of the same transfer addiction.

As much as I'd like to think I made the intentional decision to practise intuitive movement instead of rigid, ritualistic exercise, I was forced to make the decision by my body. Someone once told me that if you don't listen to your body it will force you to listen and I now know this to be true. After years of dealing with chronic pain from pushing myself too hard, horrible mood swings from not eating enough for how much I was moving and breaking my foot twice, I finally surrendered to the idea that rest, recovery and intention were more important than my Apple Watch badges. I hated taking a day off, but what was even worse was having to take months off at a time after fracturing my foot from taking too many spin classes. I realized that I was miserable without exercise and that I couldn't rely on just one tool to handle the burden of regulating my emotions, so I looked into less extreme ways to practise movement.

Instead of using movement as a tool to lose weight, look like an Instagram model or punish myself for eating, I began making the shift to focusing on how exercising made me *feel*. The first step was finding movement that brought me joy and pleasure, not pain. Maybe that should have been obvious to me from the get-go, but it wasn't. I started by going to all of my usual classes, but instead of obsessing over calorie burning, I took off the watch and allowed myself to feel the energy of the room. I signed up for classes led by instructors who motivated me with positivity and left me feeling better about myself after the session. I started taking classes that focused on recovery like Yin yoga, or restorative Pilates, and allotted myself rest days. But the most important shift I made was finding my *flow state*.

Coined by Hungarian psychologist Mihaly Csikszentmihalyi, the term "flow state" describes a mental state in which a person is entirely focused on a single task or activity and is fully in the present moment.[2] "There's this focus that leads to a sense of ecstasy, a sense of clarity: you know exactly what you want to do from one moment to the other; you get immediate feedback," Csikszentmihalyi explained in his 2004 TED Talk. During flow state, you are totally immersed in what you are doing and reach a meditative-type state. Studies have also shown that during a state of flow, your brain releases the reward neurotransmitter dopamine,[3] the same chemical messenger I'd been chasing with my drinking.

Finding my flow through intuitive movement also brought other benefits, like better performance in the exercise I was doing and less self-judgement. Letting go of my expectations allowed me to have a healthier relationship with my body, ultimately leading me to a better relationship with my inner self. A healthier relationship with myself also means I make decisions that align with my values and empower me. Now, before I work out, I ask myself *why* I am choosing to move my body and what I need on that day. If my intention is negative or punishment-based I skip the workout and use one of my mindfulness techniques to process my feelings. Exercise is no longer a weapon against my body, but a tool of self-love.

WAYS TO PRACTISE INTUITIVE MOVEMENT

Intuitive movement is a means of expressing ourselves physically without tying ourselves to exercise milestones. It's about listening to what your body really wants, rather than attempting to drown it out with booze, and it's an approach that will enable you to tune into yourself physically in any given moment. It's the complete opposite to the philosophy of "no pain, no gain!" It's not about pushing yourself to the limits, but about nourishing yourself body and soul. So what does this look like?

EMBRACE SHORT BURST MOVEMENTS

Exercise doesn't always need to take 45+ minutes; sometimes you have a full day and just don't have the time or energy. If you get the itch to move your body but you're in a crunch, a short walk outside or a mini stretching session is still beneficial to your overall health. It can also be valuable simply to focus on ten-minute increments when the mood strikes; for example, especially for those of us who work at a desk all day, just getting up and just doing some body squats or jumping jacks can improve our oxygen intake[4] and help us control our blood sugar levels.[5]

MODIFY, MODIFY, MODIFY!

If you're someone like me who enjoys group exercise, it's important to listen to your body first before following directly along with the instructor's line-up. That's not to say do your own thing, but it's crucial for your wellbeing to modify the exercise to your ability level and what is appropriate for your body. Remember that your journey is highly personal, and will look different to anyone else's. Modification is by no means a dirty word, it is just another way to gain better body awareness and avoid exercise-related injury.

FIND YOUR FLOW

There are so many different ways to move your body outside of traditional exercise or a fitness boutique. It's important you try different forms of intuitive movement so that you can find what brings you joy and keeps you in a state of flow. Some of my favourite ways to practise this involve exercises where I don't have to overthink what I'm doing, like walking, yoga at home, swimming, cycling or tai chi.

FLEXIBILITY VERSUS RIGIDITY

Similar to intuitive eating, the idea behind intuitive movement is to do it when you feel like it rather than force yourself into a structured routine. If your exercise programme is too strict and you miss a workout, you risk feeling guilty, which can lead to stress – the exact opposite of what we are trying to achieve here. Learning to be flexible, listen to your body and practise self-compassion will increase your motivation to move and ultimately improve your overall wellbeing.

LET YOUR INTUITION MOVE YOU

The beauty of intuitive movement is that it is as individual as you are. It gives you permission to work with what you have, rather than push yourself too hard or even put off exercising altogether because you worry you have to be fit or have the "perfect" body before you get started.

★ Take a moment now to reflect on how intuitive movement could feature in your own life.

★ If you already follow an exercise regime, how might intuitive movement play a role in it by allowing you to listen to your body more?

★ If you don't exercise much or at all at the moment, what sort of activity appeals to you? Walking? Pilates? Aqua aerobics? Belly dancing? Don't be afraid to think outside the box. Once you have thought of something, why not look for a class in your area?

★ How could you include intuitive movement in your routine in a way that suits you, and which helps support your soberish goals? Maybe, for example, instead of automatically heading out for a Friday night drink after work, you could join a spin class as part of your POA instead? Or if you know that you are spending the evening with friends, you could schedule an exercise session for the next morning, to make it easier to stick to your drinking goals? (Yoga with a hangover, anyone? Not to be recommended!)

DO WHAT'S RIGHT FOR YOU

"How would someone who truly loved themselves show up in this moment?" asks Lindsay Dalton – and that's the key to intuitive movement. This soberish tool offers a way to connect with your body and practise self-care on your own terms (which we will be building on in the next chapter). It allows us to act on our own internal cues to decide what type of movement, how long, and the intensity we'd like to engage in, or whether we need to rest instead.

Incorporating intuitive movement into your weekly routine as part of your POA can be a great way to prioritise other leisure activities over those that involve drinking. It can also mean it's easier to make the decision in the first place not to drink or to limit your drinking, as it's easier to say no when you know that alcohol is detrimental to physical fitness and will likely impair your performance. On top of this, intuitive movement can increase blood circulation, which makes us feel good. This natural release of dopamine may make us less inclined to turn to the unnatural release of dopamine from alcohol to cope with difficult emotions.[6]

If you are somebody who is inclined to extremes, perhaps along the lines of the binge drinker or high-risk drinker, you may find yourself diving headfirst into activities like I did, so remember that this is all about finding balance and listening to what your body really needs. There is no need to train for a marathon – unless you want to – as there is evidence to suggest that as little as five minutes of physical exercise can help to reduce alcohol cravings.[7] Most of all, have fun finding out what intuitive movement could look like for you. And when everything clicks, enjoy those moments of flow.

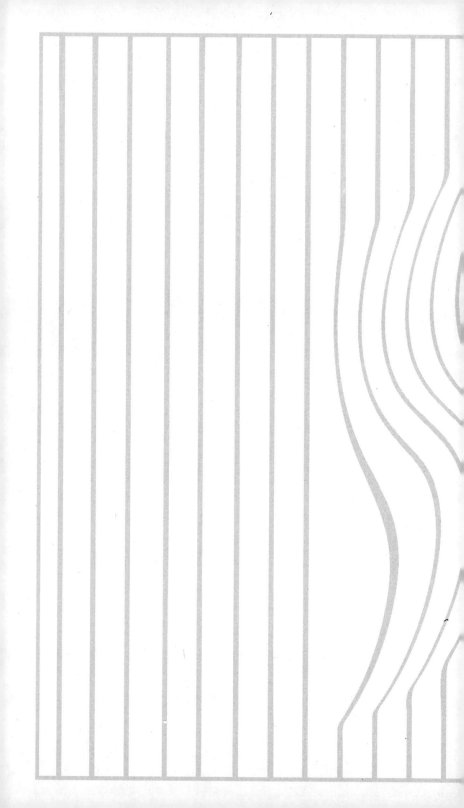

CHAPTER 8

Listen to Yourself: Develop Somatic Intuition

First off, you're probably wondering what "somatic intuition" is. You could say it's a fancy way of saying body awareness, or full-body listening. And I'm not talking about the "ouch, my arms hurt from lifting" kind of listening. Somatic intuition is about taking into account your entire body, mental, emotional state and finding the mind–body connection between these. In this respect, it builds upon a similar sort of connection that we start to create with our bodies through intuitive moment, when we tune in to what our body wants. The word "somatic" comes from the ancient Greek word *sōma*, meaning body. Somatic intuition is about connecting with yourself physically as well as mentally, but it involves asking yourself, "What is the emotional component underneath my physiological symptom?" The truth is, you've probably experienced somatic – i.e. bodily – pain or discomfort at some point in your life because of your mental or emotional state, but without even knowing it.

When I was around 13 years old I went through a stage of serious stomach issues. Severe pain in my abdominal area would occasionally cause me almost to pass out. The discomfort was unbearable at times, to the point that I would be lying on the bathroom floor, crying in a pool of sweat. My parents took me to specialists and I had my first colonoscopy, during which I had to drink barium (if you don't know what that is, I hope you never have to find out). Special X-rays were taken and nothing could be found. There was no mass or cancer, so eventually the doctors simply gave up, had me remove a few things from my diet, told me it was probably just IBS and called it a day.

Over time, I learned how to deal with the pain and used things like heating pads and magnesium supplements to decrease the discomfort. Eventually the pain dissipated, ironically enough around the time

I started drinking. But I wouldn't call it a coincidence. Looking back, after being evaluated and diagnosed properly, my hindsight is 20–20, and my stomach pain was very much a product of my severe anxiety. Throughout my entire life, I've suffered with strange phobias and mystery disorders, which could never be traced back to any physical issue. What I was really suffering from was a psychosomatic disorder – a psychological condition that leads to physical symptoms, often without any medical explanation. It can affect almost any part of the body. People who suffer from this disorder tend to seek frequent medical attention, eventually becoming frustrated because of the lack of diagnosis.[1] I was literally so stressed out from dysregulated emotions that I was making myself physically ill.

Fast-forward 17 years and I know exactly how my anxiety manifests itself in my body, the difference between muscle tension from stress and workout pain, period cramps from nervousness, and why I'm experiencing a migraine – all because I've learned full-body listening. I don't just understand my body, but have full awareness of every part of myself and what this is trying to tell me at all times. I am constantly listening to my body, and when I don't, I usually pay the price for that. If I overwork myself and don't rest or recover, my body will get fatigued and force me to; you may know this phenomenon as burnout. If I'm really stressed about a deadline or project but don't take the time to take a hot bath, go to cryotherapy or stretch, I will almost always inevitably end up with a migraine. My body is always trying to communicate with me, as is yours; the question is: *are you listening?*

SURFACE-LEVEL PROBLEMS, DEEPER ISSUES

Most of us are probably used to quieting our somatic pain with Western medicine, alcohol, drugs or food. And, yes, if you break your arm or hit your head you should absolutely see a physician. But the somatic pain I'm talking about concerns the day-to-day discomforts you feel which are brought on by unprocessed trauma and emotions. The ones you cover up with pain-relief creams, ibuprofen, yoga and massages (and I'm totally calling myself out on this one).

We all carry this kind of pain because, more often than not, we've been taught by society to cure the issue directly with medicine rather than listen to what else our body might be telling us. This may help temporarily but it doesn't solve the deeper issue. The thing about stress, pain, trauma, disappointment – we either talk about it, process it *or* we store it. It's simple science: *energy, once created, is not destroyed.*

Common forms of somatic pain caused by emotional dysregulation or trauma can include these symptoms:

* ★ stomach pain or tension
* ★ shoulder pain or tension
* ★ neck pain or tension
* ★ migraines
* ★ hair loss
* ★ acne

You can probably come up with some symptoms of your own to add to this list, which may well relate to buried emotions that you are trying to avoid through drinking.

WHAT IS YOUR BODY TRYING TO TELL YOU?

I mentioned earlier how most of us have very likely experienced somatic discomfort or outright pain at some point in our lives. I'd like to invite you to spend some time thinking about this.

★ Over the next week, stop and start to identify any potential physiological pain that comes up, such as shoulder tension or stomach pain.

★ Then think about the reasons you may be feeling somatic pain: *What emotions have I been avoiding? Am I worried? Ask yourself this "HALT" question: am I hungry, angry, lonely or tired?* As Nikita Mehta explains on page 142, HALT encourages you to pause and acknowledge what you are feeling in the moment, instead of responding to situations with a knee-jerk reaction or by falling into old habits, such as drinking.

★ Keep note of the pain and potential causes in your phone notes or in a journal.

★ After the week is over, review what you have written. Do you see any patterns? Is something stressful happening in your life that you haven't dealt with? Are you still grieving a past situation? Do you need to take a break? Would it help to speak to somebody about how you are feeling? (If you are concerned that there may be a physical cause, please do seek professional medical advice.)

★ Try asking your body what it needs and *listen*.

WHERE DO YOU HOLD YOUR STRESS?

Once you've completed the last exercise, you will probably have a much clearer idea of how repressed feelings could be trying to make themselves known to you through aches and pains in your body. So now that you know this, what should you do about it? Perhaps the answer is that you don't need to do much of anything to try to "cure" this, apart from acknowledge that it's happening and that there are reasons for this.

I tend to hold my stress in my neck and shoulders, which leads to chronic inflammation and migraines. I'm prescribed migraine medication and have a nice little pharmacy of different over-the-counter pain relief medication, numbing creams and CBD tinctures. I live a fulfilling yet exhausting lifestyle with a high-stress career as an entrepreneur, leading multiple projects, hosting podcasts, writing this book, constantly goal-setting and raising the bar for myself. People often ask me how I do everything and I can honestly say I don't know. What I do know is that it takes a toll on my body and that I have been learning over the past year how to do *less*.

After reading the book *Essentialism: The Disciplined Pursuit of Less* by Greg McKeown, I knew that the only way to sustain a successful, healthy lifestyle and also continue to pursue new goals was to take things off my plate that weren't serving my greater purpose. As someone who defines a lot of my identity through what I can accomplish, this was an extremely hard task. *If I do less, won't that make me less?* No. I realized how deep of a problem my thinking around this really was when I found myself working 70 hours per week, in the middle of a nasty separation, in a town where I knew no one and then decided I was going to become a SPENGA instructor on top of everything else, because why not, right? The anxiety of the training I was doing was causing me to have migraines almost daily. My sleep, my workouts and my mood were all suffering because I couldn't let go of becoming a SPENGA instructor.

Here's a recap of a conversation I had with myself:

Do you really need to become a SPENGA instructor?
Well, I already did the training so I *have* to commit to becoming a trainer and complete the audition process.

Why?
I've already invested time into the three-day teacher training, I can't just not do it.

Why not?
I don't know, it just isn't in my nature not to complete something.

OK, so even though the cognitive dissonance of this experience is causing you physical pain and mental breakdowns, you are going to continue because you put it on your "to-do" board? You can't just cross it out?
I mean, I guess I could. I've just never been someone who quits.

You're not quitting, Kayla, you're overcommitted. Let it go.
Crosses off SPENGA INSTRUCTOR on board – immediately feels physical and emotional relief.

In sending you messages of discomfort and pain, your body may be trying to give you a wake-up call that something isn't right. It's offering you the opportunity to stop and listen to your deeper needs. So what could you be avoiding?

PUT AVOIDANCE CENTRE-STAGE

Let's do a little exercise and see where you might be practising avoidance in your own life.

When you feel pain or discomfort in your body, instead of sitting with your emotions and allowing them to flow through you, do you opt for one of these surface-level fixes? Check off any that apply and add any of your own go-to distractions as well:

- ★ Drink alcohol
- ★ Go to the chiropractor
- ★ Get a massage
- ★ Take painkillers
- ★ Do drugs
- ★ Sweat it out

- ★ ....

- ★ ....

- ★ ....

Once you start thinking about this, you may realize that there are any number of things that you would prefer to do, rather than sit with your feelings. Some of those things may look like fun activities on a surface level, others much less so. Make a note of these too.

If you routinely practise avoidance instead of acknowledging or allowing yourself to feel your emotions, you may be operating from a "lack mentality", so let's find out more about this.

AN ABUNDANCE MINDSET

Keen to discover how adopting a different mindset can help us build better relationships with ourselves, I spoke to educator and yoga instructor Nikita Mehta, who is also a grey area drinking coach. My questions are in italic, with her answers below.

What is an abundance mindset?
An "abundance mindset" is the opposite of "lack mentality". Lack mentality says, "I have a problem and there is only one way to fix it." For many of us that was alcohol: "I am struggling with anxiety, alcohol is the way I fix it." It also gets wrapped up into our journeys afterwards: "I have a problem managing my alcohol use, complete abstinence is the only option." Lack mentality takes the fluidity and creativity out of the conversation that we are having with our own bodies.

Abundance mindset means that for anything that arises, I have an infinite amount of options on how to get my needs met. Abundance mindset means that I don't curtail my own ability to thrive.

How can you use an abundance mindset to deeply listen to your body?
Let's look at an example. It's five o'clock and you get home from work, anxiety is high and your habit is to reach for a glass of wine. Lack mentality says, "No, I will not drink that glass of wine because I don't drink anymore, but I also won't do anything else to get my

needs met." Abundance mindset says, "Let me deeply listen to my own body and figure out what my needs are and then get creative on how to meet those needs."

HALT is a great place to start in this adventure: am I hungry, angry, lonely or tired? Great, I have acknowledged that I am angry. I can spend some time accepting where that anger is coming from so that the option that I choose for myself best meets my needs. I am angry that my sister took my favourite sweater without asking. I can: 1) have a non-violent conversation with her about boundaries and permission, 2) go for a run to release excess energy or 3) take a bubble bath with essential oils.

Abundance mindset gives me the agency to listen to my body and my needs and then pick from a variety of ways to best get my needs met.

What is distress tolerance and how can we use it to create more body awareness and mind–body connection?

Distress tolerance is learning to sit in discomfort. Discomfort doesn't have to be a bad thing if we use it for its biological necessity: feedback. Our tendency so often is to dissociate with our discomfort immediately, and really we haven't been taught the skill to sit and listen to discomfort. We are so accustomed to getting discomfort out of the way as soon as possible: Does your back hurt? Here's a pill for that. Are you hungry? Press this button and the food will be delivered to your front door, you don't even need to put pants on.

In somatic intuition, we call upon distress tolerance to teach us about the mind–body connection. Not all discomforts need to be banished at once; sometimes these feedback loops are telling us that we aren't paying attention to our bodies, that we need to slow down, drink some more water, and rest longer. If we listen to discomfort, we find that it can be our greatest teacher.

At the end of the day, we need the full spectrum of emotional and physical states in order to fully feel our human life. You have to pull the pendulum back sometimes and be uncomfortable so that you know the juxtaposition of when you are feeling good and thriving. Sit in your discomfort, listen to your body, take a few breaths – nothing is stagnant; if you listen and act accordingly, real somatic relief is right around the corner. Be patient with yourself.

THE MIND-BODY FLOW

Some of us – and particularly those of us who use alcohol to self-medicate – may drink to distract ourselves from certain thoughts, stresses, memories and emotions that we would rather forget or repress. These can end up being stored by the body, which, despite our conscious best efforts, may continue communicating them to us through means such as aches and pains and illness, so that they can eventually be released and tackled. During the course of your soberish journey, include the tool of somatic intuition in your POA as a way to acknowledge and express potentially buried emotions.

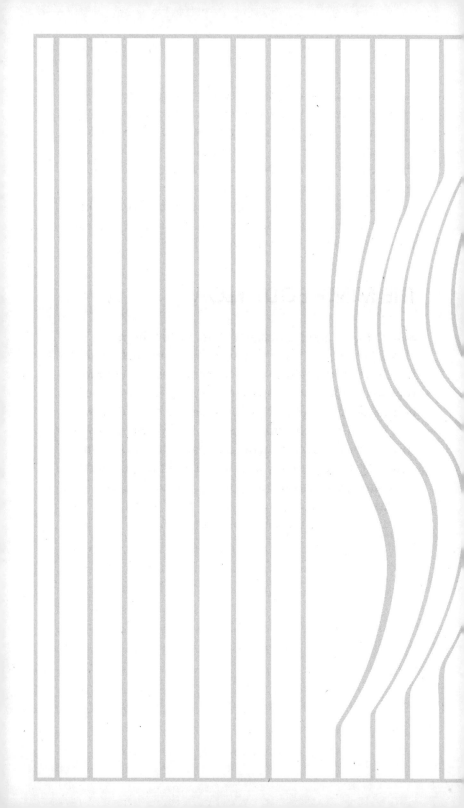

CHAPTER 9

Chill Out: Cold Exposure Therapy

The first time I was introduced to cold exposure was through a therapist who was helping me learn how to cope with my panic attacks without using drugs. The reason I ever got started on benzodiazepines (drugs like klonopin, valium and xanax) was because I was suffering from panic disorder and could barely leave the house. I had basically become a shell of a person. Fast-forward five years and I was heavily addicted to klonopin and also abusing alcohol to self-medicate. My anxiety was so severe I really couldn't make it more than a day or two without drinking or using my pills. I hated the way I was living, but not having alcohol or my pills scared me even more than continuing to lose friends and watch my life spiral out of control. And so the cycle continued – until that fateful moment when I realized I had to stop or I was going to end up another statistic of Big Pharma and Big Alcohol.

I've been using different forms of cold exposure therapy for the past seven years and it is still one of the most effective tools (in my opinion) for grounding myself and releasing uncomfortable emotions instead of avoiding them by using alcohol or pills. When I'm experiencing severe anxiety or panic attacks in situations like driving alone or being in crowded spaces, my body tends to go into fight-or-flight mode, with rapid heartbeats, hot flashes, tunnel vision and an acute sense of doom. Not fun. All of this is happening because of old triggers telling me that I'm not safe – and so my body jumps into action to try to protect me.

To ground myself in these moments, I use ice to help jolt my system out of this mode. The ice helps me to focus on the physical sensation of the cold rather than the negative sensations happening because of my anxiety. To this day, I carry an ice pack or a bag of ice with me pretty much everywhere I go. When available and when my negative emotions are more overwhelming, I've also used cold showers in these moments. It's helpful for me to know I can turn to a tangible tool that has effectively worked for me for years. Over time, I have tried higher levels of cold exposure through cryotherapy and ice baths. Both forms have been extremely beneficial in helping me regulate my emotions on a deeper level, face my fears, test my mental strength and improve my physical health.

LET'S TALK ICE-COLD BENEFITS

According to Andrew Huberman, Professor of Neurobiology and Ophthalmology at Stanford School of Medicine and host of the Huberman Lab podcast (one of my favourites), deliberately exposing yourself to cold for just 11 minutes per week can help you achieve the benefits of cold exposure. This could be distributed throughout the week in 1–5-minute increments using any of the methods I mentioned earlier and which I'm also going to be inviting you to try later on in this chapter. (No need to shiver; it'll be fine, I promise!) There are many different mental and emotional benefits of cold exposure. These include the following:

REDUCES SYMPTOMS OF DEPRESSION

Research has shown a correlation between those with depression and higher levels of inflammation in their bodies. The dysregulation that inflammation can cause in your body, like suppressing your immune system, can directly affect the way you respond to treatment like anti-depressants.[1] Even if you don't currently suffer or have a history of depression, inflammation can make you more susceptible to depression.[2] Inflammation in the body is a direct response to something that your immune system deems an irritant. (And yes, besides being a depressant in its own right, alcohol can be one of these irritants, especially when it comes to its effect on the gut.)[3] Symptoms can include pain, redness, heat, swelling or general discomfort.[4] Normally we think of inflammation as being caused by something physical like exercise, or something foreign like a virus, but inflammation can also be our body's response to stress. Have you ever experienced neck or shoulder pain because of stress? Migraines or tension headaches? These are perfect examples of our body trying to tell us something; however, as we saw in chapter 8, we usually just don't listen or we use surface-level fixes like over-the-counter pain relievers or anti-inflammatories. The Wim Hof Method, in which breathing exercises and cold exposure are paired together, has been scientifically proven to suppress inflammation as well as improve sleep and decrease stress.[5] (We'll be diving deeper into the Wim Hof Method soon with a short interview with Marcus Bradley, a level-two Wim Hof Method Instructor.)

RELEASES NEUROCHEMICALS

We looked at neurochemicals in Part One, but let's revisit their importance. Did you know that deliberately exposing yourself to the cold releases both epinephrine (adrenaline) and norepinephrine, a neurotransmitter made up of dopamine?[6] At first, the release of these two neurochemicals can make us feel uncomfortable, and tell us to "get out!" This is where we need to practise mental strength and fight the urge to step out of the cold. Through this exposure, we stand to gain increased levels of energy and focus that can be lasting and as effective as a cup of coffee. Cold exposure also releases one of our favourite neurotransmitters:

dopamine, the pleasure chemical! Using cold exposure like cold showers, cryotherapy and cold baths causes the prolonged release of dopamine.[7]

INCREASES HAPPINESS LEVELS AND REGULATES EMOTIONS

We'll look more closely at different ways to increase your overall happiness and wellbeing in chapter 16, but cold exposure is a great place to start. Using the Wim Hof Method for breathing and cold exposure, you can learn to develop and find your own sense of happiness, which you may have lost to some degree through alcohol. Learning proper breathwork techniques can play a huge role in helping us learn to control and regulate our minds. Controlled breathing exercises, like the ones you will be learning in chapter 10 of this book, can help you activate your parasympathetic nervous system (PSNS), relieve stress and make you feel more comfortable. Proper and deliberate breathing can influence and control your emotions, allowing you to take your power back and increase your happiness.[8] The same way in which cold exposure can decrease symptoms of depression, it allows for the increase of dopamine transmissions in the neural pathways, boosting your mood naturally.[9]

WORKOUT RECOVERY

If you already exercise regularly, or plan on adding intuitive movement into your practice, it's important to allow your body to recover from physical exercise. Every time you exercise, your body is depleted of energy and temporarily damages muscular tissue to allow for muscle growth. This means you need to allow time for your body to rest and recover in order to avoid injuries, inflammation or delayed-onset muscle soreness (DOMS). Coupled with our other tools of proper nutrition and sleep hygiene, cold exposure can be extremely beneficial for workout recovery as it reduces inflammation and muscle soreness caused by exercise.[10] It also allows for better sleep, which means more time for your body to rest and restore itself.

REDUCES BLOOD PRESSURE

As someone aged 30 who suffers from high blood pressure, with no history of obesity or smoking, who exercises regularly and has been in recovery from AUD for almost seven years, this benefit was a big one for me. If I run down the list of things that cause high blood pressure, I don't check any of them except one: STRESS. I take an SNRI for my OCD, medication to help me sleep and hormonal birth control, so the last thing I want to do is throw a high blood pressure pill into the mix if I can avoid it. By practising cold exposure and breathing techniques I'm working on lowering my blood pressure. Practising consistently helps lower your heart rate, strengthen your immune system alongside the absorption of nutrients and oxygen into your cells more effectively.[11]

IMMUNITY BOOSTER

A weak immune system can lead you to be more susceptible to viruses and diseases, so a healthy system is vital for your overall health. As we mentioned earlier, a suppressed immune system can also negatively impact our mental health. Managing our stress is a big part of keeping both our immune system and our blood pressure in check. As you will discover in chapter 10, breathwork is a powerful stress-reducer, as well as a way to maintain low levels of stress on a regular basis. Exposing yourself to the cold and practising a short breathwork each day can help strengthen your immune system.

IMPROVED METABOLISM

Having proper metabolism is important for a plethora of reasons; good gut health, serotonin production and of course the production of food into fuel. Metabolism allows for our body to make food into energy that we use for essential functions.[12] Some of our basic metabolic functions include:

- ★ breathing
- ★ circulating blood
- ★ digesting food
- ★ growing and repairing cells
- ★ managing hormone levels
- ★ regulating body temperature

Cold exposure is a great way for us to force our bodies to produce heat through the response of shivering. Shivering generates heat, which helps the body improve its metabolism in a natural way. Exposing the body to the cold on a safe and regular basis can increase the metabolic rate by about 16 per cent.[13] If all of the above still hasn't persuaded you of the benefits of cold therapy, perhaps hearing it directly from an expert will!

A CONVERSATION ABOUT COLD TREATMENTS

I spoke with Marcus Bradley, a level-two Wim Hof Method instructor, to ask him about his work and about the benefits of cold therapy. Here's what he said:

What is your personal definition of cold exposure and breathwork? What is the connection?

Cold exposure is a method of putting ourselves in an uncomfortable, controlled stress to ultimately reap physical and mental benefits. This is done by exposing ourselves to cold conditions like ice baths, cold showers, cryotherapy, or "ocean dunking" (immersion in water that is under 15°C/59°F). Breathwork is a form of calming stress by focusing on the breath, which can be done in a number of ways. Mainly by diaphragm breathing and activating the PSNS. It can also be a tool to use for meditation. Breathwork is a way of priming the body to deal with stress and cold therapy/exposure is that stress. [Cold therapy] is a controlled stress test where we can use our breathwork to help us activate the PSNS.

How can an individual use cold therapy/exposure to improve their mental health and overall wellbeing?

The simple act of a cold shower can improve your mental health and wellbeing by giving you more energy, improving metabolism through eustress [a form of beneficial stress], immunity boosters and naturally floods your body with dopamine and endorphins. Starting the day off with something tough gives mental clarity and focus: I've already accomplished something for the day, probably the most difficult thing I'll have to do, which makes the rest of the day seem easier. It provides a zest for life. It gives more confidence because I can walk into a room and know I have done something most people don't imagine they are capable of doing. It's not that they can't, but they've never allowed themselves to get to that level of discomfort. On days when I'm depressed, exposing myself to the cold is an immediate game-changer. It's the exact 180 of drinking: I thought drinking would give me relief when in reality it gives me short-term relief, then short- and long-term consequences and pain. With cold exposure, it's a few minutes of discomfort for an entire day of enhanced mood, confidence and energy.

Anything else you feel is important to add?
People tend to think taking an ice bath is scary. With that in mind, it's just that concept of how powerful our minds are and how it's always seeking comfort, whether it be through distractions, or overeating, or drinking, we are constantly numbing ourselves so we don't have to feel. When we get into the cold water we are forced to feel everything. That feeling and the surrender to the feeling is that first light-bulb moment that all my clients get of "wow, this isn't as bad as I thought it was," similar to what you experienced. Once you do that with something like an ice bath, that is very tough and raw. You start asking yourself what else is there that I think is a big deal and probably isn't anymore. The ice bath and winning that mental battle can really jump-start a lot of things for people in a big way.

READY TO GIVE IT A TRY?

You don't have to take yourself off to an icy ocean and submerge yourself in the freezing waters to experience the benefits of cold exposure. Why not start small by giving one of the following exercises a go?

THE ICE CUBE HACK

One of the first techniques my therapist taught me was the ice cube hack, which I now use as a form of instant first aid. It can be quite uncomfortable to hold ice cubes, which helps your neurotransmitters to refocus on the pain coming from the cold rather than the feelings of panic.

★ This technique works by holding ice cubes or an ice pack in your hands, on your neck or close to your chest. (I personally like to hold the ice cubes in my hands or put an icepack on the back of my neck.)

★ For ice packs, 10 minutes' exposure should be long enough. For ice cubes, make the time shorter and move the ice about a little so that it doesn't stick to your skin. Always pay close attention to how your skin feels to avoid ice burn.

★ To avoid ice burn, remember the acronym CBAN: cold, burn, ache and numb. As soon as you feel any numbness, remove the ice.[14]

This can be a handy little tool to have in your POA kit whenever you find yourself feeling anxious at social functions or about to lose your temper in a heated moment. Just take yourself somewhere quiet for a moment with a tumbler of ice and give yourself time to cool down until you feel ready to return to the situation.

30-DAY COLD SHOWER CHALLENGE

Yup, this one is exactly what it sounds like! Commit to 30 consecutive days of taking a cold shower. You can do this one of two ways as a beginner: contrast showers or ending your showers with cold water. Contrast showers use cold exposure through alternating between warm and cold water.

* ★ Start with warm water and then turn your shower to the coldest setting you can handle for 15 to 30 seconds, then go back to warm. Continue to alternate.
* ★ The goal here is to increase your tolerance to the cold, so that you need shorter periods of warm water in between the cold.
* ★ The second way is by taking your shower as normal and ending the shower with the coldest setting for 15 to 30 seconds.
* ★ Work your way up to two minutes of cold water exposure by the end of the 30 days.

• •

WATER BOWL PLUNGE

Again, this one is pretty self-explanatory!

* ★ Take a large salad or mixing bowl and fill it up with cold water and ice.
* ★ Insert both your hands, feet or face for up to one minute.
* ★ This will feel uncomfortable, but that's the point. In order for us to face our fears and negative emotions we must get uncomfortable.

• •

If cold treatments appeal and you want to take it further, you could discover that cold-water swimming is the way to go for you.[15]

KEEP IT COOL

Cold exposure has been proven to have incredible benefits for treating depression and health conditions caused by inflammation in the body. While deliberately getting cold is something that most of us avoid at all costs, it's definitely worth considering adding this one to your soberish toolkit. If you tend to be a boredom drinker, why not wake up with a bang in the form of a cold shower? It could give you a euphoric hit of adrenaline and a sense of achievement to start your day. Or, if you are inclined to go all-out for things, in the way that binge drinkers often do, maybe challenge yourself to make the water bowl plunge part of your POA for a set period of time, and keep a note of the benefits during and afterwards.

As we touched on earlier, cold exposure therapy can have even more impact when combined with forms of breathwork, as this will help you to still your mind and focus in the cold. In fact, whatever the circumstances, breathwork and meditation are both extremely helpful practices, which is why we are going to be exploring them next.

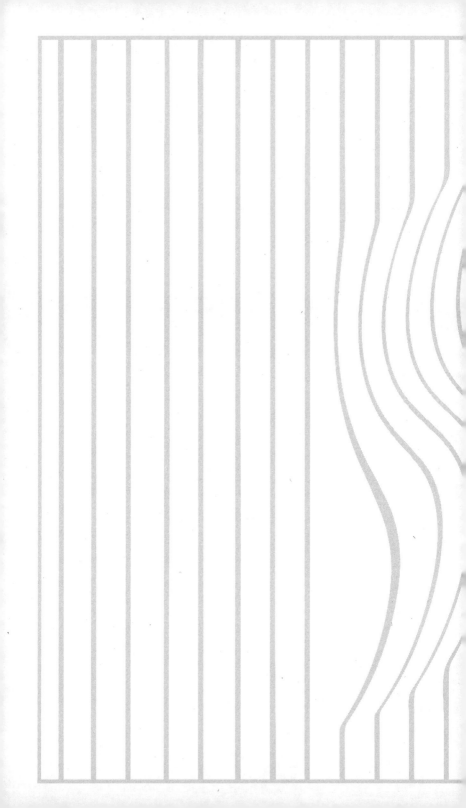

CHAPTER 10

Turn Inward: Breathwork and Meditation

Meditation has been a huge propellant in my own healing journey. I started my meditation practice after leaving AA, when I felt I needed something to replace the meetings and commitments I was no longer attending. I also needed to find a deeper connection to myself and my trauma, which I hadn't experienced in "the rooms". I tried a few different meditation apps before I landed on one that particularly spoke to me. It may have been the way I connected to the voice of my guide, but I found it was a lot easier to have a steady practice if the person I was listening to made me feel at peace. For me, this was Andy of the Headspace app.

I found guided meditation the easiest way to start my practice. It was passive, so all I had to do was sit in a comfortable position and listen for 10 to 15 minutes, and do whatever my guide told me to. Sometimes that meant a guided visualization or a body scan and other times it was simply silence. Those silent sessions seemed to be the toughest meditations for me at first. I would avoid them if possible; that was until, unbeknownst to me, I signed up for one in person.

Every week, the yoga studio I attend holds 30-minute meditation classes and I decided to go along to one. I hadn't been to an in-person meditation session before, but I assumed it would be similar to what I did at home: sit comfortably, close my eyes and listen to my guide. Unfortunately, I was very wrong. I walked in, sat down and put a light blanket over myself in preparation for the next 30 minutes. The teacher sat down and began the class, only to announce that this would be a silent meditation. "Ah, what the fuck!" was literally the first thing that came to my mind. I wasn't sure why at the time, but my immediate reaction to this was *fear*. The idea of sitting with my own thoughts, or whatever else was roaming up there, for 30 whole minutes sounded disastrous and I felt anxiety creep up my spine. I wanted to get up and walk out of the room, but instead I put into action what I had been learning from Andy. I sat in the feeling and it slowly dissipated.

For the next 30 minutes, I remained in silence, repeating in my thoughts the "Om" mantra we'd been given. And I allowed myself to feel everything I had been avoiding, which was a lot. I had just unwillingly relocated across the country to move in with my parents after going through a messy separation, and I'd also quit a very toxic work environment, leaving me jobless. I felt as though everything around me was burning to the ground and all that was left was a pile of ash. I was heart-broken, angry, resentful, disappointed and lonely. All I wanted to do was scream or cry or sleep, but I knew that wasn't going to help me grieve or heal; so here I was, sitting in a silent meditation class, feeling it all.

That's when it hit me. *I am feeling all of this.* It felt like every prickly pear cactus inside me was pulsating, and yet I didn't shut the feelings down or immediately leave and head to the bar across the street. My fears hadn't just surfaced, they were real, but I was facing them instead of numbing them with alcohol. At that moment, I realized I wasn't crying because my life was in shambles; I was crying because, despite being surrounded by ash, I was practising acceptance, I was healing.

This experience, and others like it, is the reason meditation can be so important when changing your relationship with alcohol. As Lindsay Dalton, trauma-informed breathwork facilitator, tells me when we meet: "Meditation is learning to sit and listen to your internal experience. By doing so you strengthen your practice like a muscle and over time this seeps into so many other areas of your life." When you first take alcohol out of the picture as a device for dealing with your uncomfortable emotions, you may be unsure how to regulate those feelings. Through meditation you can become more in tune with your emotions, gain a greater sense of self-control and find a sense of inner peace.

And if you're intimidated by the idea of meditation, you aren't alone. "People are afraid they are going to do it wrong, or that they need to spend a ton of time on meditation to have a practice," says Lindsay, "but there is no wrong way to experience meditation. Every session serves a purpose. You can practise for as little as three to five minutes a day using a timer and see results."

BREATHWORK

The breath sits at the heart of many different types of meditation. "Your breath is your home base," explains Lindsay. "As your anchor to the present moment, it is a vital part of meditation. When used consistently and therapeutically, it can also aid in your journey of healing from past trauma by connecting the conscious and unconscious mind." As a powerful tool for nervous system regulation, conscious connected breathing – also known as breathwork – stimulates the parasympathetic nervous system. This sends a signal to our brain that helps us access a safe, calm and relaxed state, so we can let go of any of the four trauma responses that might surface in moments of stress: fight, flight, freeze or fawn. As mentioned earlier, in the POA example given on pages 87–9, breathwork can be a helpful tool to include in your

POA as it can be a way to calm down both before and during the sorts of stressful situations that may otherwise prompt you to drink. Breathwork also pulls more oxygen into your system, allowing your muscles to relax and your mind to think more clearly.[1] When you practise holding your breath for short periods, CO_2 levels in your blood increase, which in turn increases the cardio-inhibitory response that lowers your heart rate.[2]

The following exercises will introduce you to three types of breathwork. If at any point you start to feel anxious or short of breath during them, simply stop the exercise and return to your normal pattern of breathing. There is absolutely no need to force anything – just let it flow.

BOX BREATHING

Also known as square breathing, box breathing is a deep-breathing technique that can clear your mind and slow down your heart rate. But make sure you don't end up overdoing it, or counting too quickly, as you could end up panting! If four seconds feels too long, you can start with two or three seconds.

- ★ Breathe in calmly for four counts.
- ★ Hold for four counts.
- ★ Exhale for four counts
- ★ Hold for four counts before repeating.
- ★ Repeat for three to four cycles.

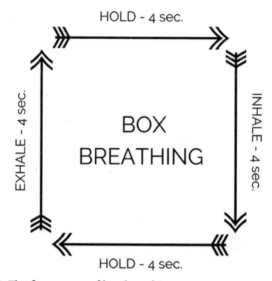

Figure 5. The four stages of box breathing.

● ●

4-7-8

While based in Pranayama, an ancient breath technique that originates from yogic practices, this form of breathwork was developed in the West by Dr Andrew Weil. He refers to it as a "natural tranquilizer for the nervous system".[3]

- ★ Breathe in for four counts.
- ★ Hold that breath for seven counts.
- ★ Now, exhale for eight counts.
- ★ Repeat until you begin to feel your heart rate slow down, your body relax and your nervous system return to a normal state.

● ●

LADDER BREATHING

This technique can seem a little trickier than other breathing techniques in your toolkit but it's extremely efficient in turning on your parasympathetic nervous system (PSNS), which tells you that you can relax. It's also great for strengthening our mindfulness, as we need to be present and pay close attention to what we are doing during our soberish journey, so that we don't fall back into harmful old habits and instead create rewarding new ones. As Wim Hoff instructor Marcus Bradley explains it:

★ Begin by getting into a comfortable seated position with your back straight, and with one hand over your heart and the other over your stomach.

★ Once you are in a comfortable position, start by breathing deep in through the nose, then breathe out through the mouth seven times. The key here is to focus on the number, so make sure to count your breath: *"in, one, out, one; in, two, out two . . ."* until you've reached seven.

★ Then you begin again, this time taking 14 breaths. Continue in increments of seven until you reach 28. If you mess up, or over-count, start again from the beginning.

MEDITATION

While I personally practise guided meditation and more recently silent meditation, there are many ways to meditate. The point isn't how you do it, but how you experience it. "Meditation is about becoming the observer of your internal experience," explains Lindsay. "The key is to simply practise by doing. Paying attention to what thoughts and emotions are surfacing, in a loving and non-judgemental way." Through trial and error, and some experimentation, you will find a type of meditation that suits you; it could be as simple as a form of breathwork or as complicated as some types of extended visualization techniques. No type of meditation is considered "better" than another; the key thing is whether it works for you. This can be an especially great tool to include in your POA if you are somebody who is prone to stress or anxiety. Over the next few pages are a couple of exercises to get you started.

MINDFULNESS MEDITATION

Because of its simple nature, this style of meditation is a great place for beginners to dip their toes into a meditative practice.

★ Turn off devices and make sure you are sitting comfortably. If you wish, you can close your eyes.

★ Now just follow and focus on the natural flow and sensation of the breath entering and leaving your body.

★ Keep returning to this sensation of the breath over and over again whenever the mind wanders and gets lost in thought. Allow any thoughts to float past like clouds.

★ Thoughts surface, return to the breath; thoughts surface, return to the breath; thoughts surface, return to the breath, and repeat . . .

★ Start by focusing like this for five minutes, gradually building up to sessions of 20 minutes.

It can be easy to overcomplicate this form of meditation, but it is truly that simple. With practise, you will be surprised at how therapeutic this process can become and how long you can actually sit and just *be*.

MOVEMENT MEDITATION

This is exactly what it sounds like. Yoga isn't the only way to practise movement meditation; there is also walking, gardening and tai chi. Movement meditation gives you an opportunity to ground yourself while simultaneously being a sponge to your environment.

★ A simple way to begin this practice would be by taking a 10-minute nature walk.

★ Walk slowly while concentrating on what you can see, hear and feel.

★ If walking doesn't appeal to you, try planting something in your garden or in a container, while focusing on the touch of the soil, the smells and sounds around you.

★ If your thoughts start wandering to your to-do list or other distractions, keep bringing your focus back to what you are doing and your surroundings – the sensations of touch, sight, sound, hearing, the ground beneath your feet.

Movement meditation is a great starting point for those looking to develop body awareness and gain a conscious connection to their body. Body awareness is important in our soberish journey because it allows us to recognize our emotional and physical cues more easily. If we're more conscious of how we are feeling, we'll be better able to identify our triggers and beat the craving – maybe even through doing a practice like movement meditation.

MANTRA-BASED MEDITATION (MBM)

A mantra can be a word or a phrase that you repeat while practising breathwork. Research has shown that mantra-based meditation (MBM) produces significant small to moderate reductions in levels of anxiety and stress (including post-traumatic stress) in those who practise it, as well as small but also significant improvements in depression and mental health-related quality of life. Other outcomes (i.e., burnout, insomnia, substance consumption) also have shown improvements.[4]

My favourite ways to practise this type of meditation are with "I am" statements like "I am worthy of the gifts the universe brings me," or simply, "I am confident." "I am" is a declaration of being. It is so powerful because it allows you to break down walls you have built inside and connect with your true self.

★ Take a moment now to write down a couple of statements like this; for example: "I am powerful", "I am able", "I am valued", "I am successful".

★ Sit or stand in front of a mirror and repeat one of these back to yourself a number of times.

★ Be aware of any resistance that comes up: you may feel awkward or even like a fraud at first, but keep going – you are re-educating your brain.

MBM is a powerful tool for overcoming negative thinking. "Your brain doesn't know the difference between what you are telling it or thinking and what you are actually experiencing," explains Lindsay. Which makes a lot of sense. A great example would be the power of anxiety. You can feel anxious in anticipation of a future event or a perceived outcome and you may experience a stress response such as an elevated heart rate, even though nothing has actually happened. When we flip the script with positive mantras like "I am capable" or "I am confident", we are re-educating our brain to believe these statements. We can even increase our level of optimism through using positive affirmations in MBM.[5] Not only can they help improve your self-esteem in the long term, and help you tackle the emotions that may prompt you to drink in that way, but mantras are a supportive tool to draw on if you are about to enter a potentially stressful situation, like a job interview, exam or an encounter with somebody who might not be as supportive of your soberish journey as you'd like them to be.

BREATHE IN THE MOMENT

In a world that places so much value on busyness and doing, it may seem counterintuitive to find that there are so many benefits to be had from just taking a moment to sit and breathe. Maybe think of breathwork and meditation as being like pressing "reset" on your body and mind: when we pause and breathe deeply and slowly, we are telling our brains that everything is OK. We are in no immediate danger and we can take a break right now from the tangle of everyday thoughts that cause stress and anxiety. And then we can recalibrate ourselves so that life generally seems more manageable and there is less temptation for us to rely on potentially harmful props like alcohol. Instead, we have a whole range of other tools that we can turn to, another of which is closely linked to meditation and equally simple yet effective: sound healing, which we are going to be looking at next.

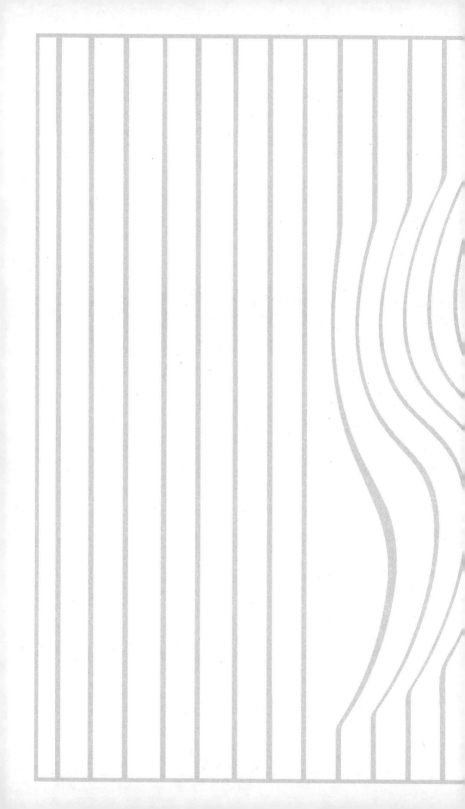

CHAPTER 11

Tune In:
Sound Healing

One of the simplest yet most effective tools you can reach for when you are feeling overstimulated is sound healing. Sound healing allows your brain to decompress while simultaneously turning on your parasympathetic nervous system. And the best part about it? You don't have to do anything but listen.

My first experience with sound healing was when I attended a sound bath with a friend, in support of another friend who was serving non-alcoholic cocktails at the event. I really wasn't sure how I felt about attending a sound bath, as it sounded a little silly (yes, even for me, a crystal-toting, vision-boarding Californian). But I wanted to keep an open mind because I also never thought I would be someone who purchased crystals or drank green juice and woke up early on Sundays without a hungover. So there I was, and I'm honestly so grateful I attended, because what I experienced can only be described as something close to flow state. I left afterwards feeling lighter, calmer and completely refreshed, as if someone had plugged me in and fully charged my Body Battery (see page 231). I knew immediately that I had found another tool to add to my soberish toolkit.

Not only does sound healing allow your mind to decompress, "It builds resilience, reduces stress and allows you to reprocess negative emotions and release them," says Farzana Ali, a brilliant UK sound therapist and author. "Sound healing works by slowing down brain-wave activity, a process called sympathetic resonance," she tells me when we speak on Zoom, "which allows for you to rest, reflect and relax."[1] The specific brain-wave activity she referred to is called alpha brain-wave activity, which is dominant when we are in a state of relaxation.[2] In layman's terms, when we practise sound healing our body and brain lower in resonant frequency, bringing us closer to our natural state of rest.

"This lower frequency and alignment of vibration slows down our brain activity to match the sound wave, which signals to our bodies we are in a safe place," explains Farzana. "Everything we do is about safety and replicating a place of rest. When we use sound healing or sound therapy we are activating our parasympathetic nervous system, which is a network in our body that relaxes us after a period of stress. Once the parasympathetic system is activated our brain goes into active recovery. This is when we increase our joy, resilience and our ability to see things from a more positive perspective."

Which all makes perfect sense if you think about it. At one point in history, our ancestors were busy running away from sabre-tooth tigers and hunting and gathering while constantly watching out for danger. For them, being in fight-or-flight mode was a necessity at all times. With the exception of those living in very dangerous circumstances, most of us luckily don't have that kind of problem anymore, but this doesn't stop our brain from thinking we do. That's why it's crucial we practise activities that bring us to a state of rest and relaxation as part of our soberish journey. Otherwise we may become anxious, highly strung and stressed out, which can lead to mental illness, high blood pressure and even heart disease.[3]

"Different sound vibrations interact with our physical and energetic bodies in beneficial ways," Summer Muse emails me on another occasion.[4] She is the amazing sound healer I had the pleasure of experiencing my first sound bath with. She adds, "Sound travels about four times faster through water than it does through air. Because our human bodies are about 70 per cent water, sound can easily recalibrate our whole system."

The benefits of sound healing have been shown to include the following:

* activates higher states of consciousness
* increases awareness and concentration
* unlocks blocked emotions
* decreases depression
* normalizes blood pressure
* relieves physical pain
* releases emotional trauma

What's not to like?

GETTING STARTED WITH SOUND HEALING

We don't always have the time or resources to go to a spa, take a day off or go to the gym, which is why it's important we have tools in our soberish toolkit and POA that work quickly, effectively and with little to no effort or cost. So where do we start when it comes to sound healing?

"One of the easiest ways to engage in sound healing is to simply go outside and engage in nature. All you need is five minutes. This could be listening to the leaves rustling in the trees, the birds singing their songs or the crash of an ocean wave," says Farzana. "If you don't have access to nature, perhaps you live in a city, you can look up alpha brain wave songs or meditations on free channels like YouTube or Spotify." (One of my personal favourites is The Sound Bath channel on Spotify.)

Turn on a meditation or alpha brain-wave channel of your choice on a streaming platform, where you can even find sound bath ceremonies for working with specific emotions, chakras and healing intentions. When it comes to tuning in, do whatever feels right for you. You will likely benefit from as little as five minutes. Summer Muse explains:

> A rule I live by is the 5x5 rule – if it doesn't matter in five years, don't spend more than five minutes being upset by it. If and when you feel a moment of discouragement, remember this, and what you have control over. Responding with a positive by turning on sound therapy and sitting in stillness will do wonders for five minutes out of your day.
>
> Let everything flow through you, and then when those five minutes are up, open your eyes, and ask yourself if you still want to feel that craving or emotion. It's not a replacement to your habits, but a redirection to create better ones – that add value and allow you to have some introspection. Combining breathwork during these moments is an additional bonus! Our bodies have the power to heal themselves, if we desire to tap within. Use your words. Use your breath. Use your sound. Let the process dance with you. It is an act of love.

If you do happen to have a bit more time, another way to engage in sound healing is through sound therapy. "Sound therapy is a more specific sound treatment used to reprocess negative emotions and release them. It is more detailed and pertains to a specific problem," explains Farzana.

A good example of sound therapy would be attending a sound bath. "A sound bath is a meditative acoustic sound concert that 'washes' away stress and brings you to a state of relaxation, activating your body's own natural system of self-healing. It is a wellness practice to tap into being present," Summer tells me.

You can find local sound baths by looking them up through Eventbrite, MeetUp.com or calling your local wellness/yoga centre. Attending sound baths can also be beneficial to building community. When you're exploring a new relationship with alcohol, sometimes those around us aren't as supportive as we'd like them to be or we realize some of our relationships are solely based around drinking. Sound baths can be a great place to find others who are on a similar pathway to healing and creating a healthier lifestyle. This will open up your social circle to new friends and a potential new support system – another of the tools that we will be looking at.

SOUND OUT HOW YOU FEEL

If you can't get outdoors to listen to nature, or attend a sound bath in person, and if you'd like some RL alternatives, you can try these simple techniques:

• •

HUMMING

Also called *bhramari pranayama* (*bhramari* is derived from the Sanskrit word for bee), this can increase the nitric oxide in your body,[5] allowing for better blood flow and in this way relaxing your nervous system.

- ★ Sit comfortably and take a moment or two to settle down. Allow your eyes to close.
- ★ Take a couple of relaxed breaths.
- ★ Inhale and, keeping your facial muscles relaxed, make a moderately loud buzzing noise while exhaling with your teeth slightly separated.

★ Let the sound fill your whole head. (If you wish, you can press gently with your index fingers on the bump of cartilage next to your ears to block them.)

★ Repeat the cycle six times before opening your eyes.

. . . .

SIGH IT OUT

I love breathwork, which is why I've included guidance on it on pages 162–5. Taking a moment to be still and tune in to your breathing can be an easy yet powerful way to find calm and let go of repressed feelings safely and constructively. When working with sound, you can combine breathwork with releasing pent-up emotions through sighs to activate your vagus nerve, the main component of the parasympathetic nervous system.

★ Cyclic sighing is exhale-focused, which means that the exhalation takes twice as long as the inhalation.

★ Inhale two short breaths through the nose.

★ Exhale in one long, sighing breath through the mouth.

★ Repeat for a couple of minutes, building up to five minutes over time.

. . . .

TAP INTO YOUR INNER CHILD

Your inner child is the childlike aspect of yourself that lives on in you. This aspect of yourself contains a lot of emotions from the past, particularly from when you were growing up, as well as your childhood dreams for the future. You can work with your inner child in all sorts of ways, but an easy practice is by giving yourself permission to play and express energy and emotions in the way you likely did without thinking as a kid.

★ Take some time out of your week to allow your inner child to make some noise.

★ This is all about being as childlike and silly as you like, so put on some sounds and jump around!

★ Enjoy dancing, hollering and releasing those blocked prickly pears of accumulated hurt and negativity through the power of expression.

★ If you like, you can play with instruments, and/ or use your body as one! (Air guitar, anybody?)

★ Go wild and let your inner child free!

MAKE SOME NOISE

Sound healing works on the level of pure energy and its vibrations; even if we can't hear well, sound waves can move through our bodies and affect us physically. As Summer Muse explains:

> We have the power to heal ourselves – everything we need is found within, and that includes our voice, our words, our affirmations. It is extremely important to remember that our words are energy; our thoughts guide us into a process that defines our beliefs and reality. Speaking kindly to ourselves is crucial in self-healing because even when you're joking, your body doesn't know the difference. In turn, a frequency is released that can raise your vibration or lower your vibration.

We all have the power to make some noise – for good or bad – so why not use sound as a way to introduce some harmony into your life? Whatever your drinking habits or your usual taste in music, sound healing can be a great tool to include in your POA to bring some calming vibes into your weekly routine. And if you'd like to balance sound therapies with a quieter activity, you can always try journaling, which we're going to look at next.

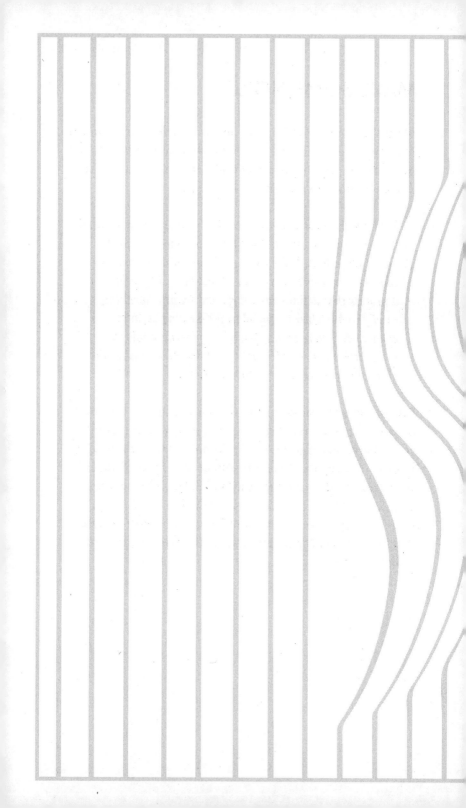

CHAPTER 12

Write It Out: Journaling

I'll be honest, this tool was one of the hardest for me to get into. Even as a writer, there was something about journaling that I was hesitant about – probably the fact that there was no instant gratification involved. Go figure! So many of my friends raved about their experience with journaling that I bought a bunch of different kinds to see which one spoke to me, but I still really struggled in the beginning to stick with it.

What really changed my mind about the entire process was learning about how much science-based evidence there was behind how journaling can help you improve your mental health, increase your performance, navigate better decision-making and help you achieve your goals.[1] Journaling is about so much more than just writing down how your day went, like in a traditional diary; it can be broken down into different categories that serve specific purposes, like increasing your gratitude or recognizing your behaviour patterns. Soberish grapevine member Claire puts it this way:

> I started journaling a couple years ago because I felt kind of lost and I wanted to reconnect with myself. I was trying to moderate alcohol at the time I started my journal and I would often write about the times that I drank (my motivations and feelings before, during, and after the drink). I was really trying to be "mindfully sober", which to me at the time meant that I was drinking but was aware of the effect that the drinks had on me and overly aware of how frequently I was drinking. I was soberish for a couple years before I went fully sober. My relationship with alcohol is something I often process and reflect on in my journals. When I was drinking, writing about it was a way to keep myself accountable. It's exciting to see the growth in my sobriety throughout the pages of my journals.

I spoke with the wider soberish community about their favourite forms of journaling and the top five most popular include free writing, gratitude lists, bullet journaling, dream journaling and reflection journaling, so let's look at these in a little more detail.

FREE WRITING

The idea behind free writing is to write for a certain length of time or to fill a specific number of pages without stopping until your timer runs out or the pages are full. It doesn't matter what you write about, the only "rule" is that you have to do so without stopping or judging what you write.

This kind of journaling can help you better understand the problems you're going through and practise goalsetting around the issue. It also creates a safe place in which to analyse your thoughts and address these without judgement. This may seem simplistic, but the idea is that if you can learn to accept what you write without judgement, you can learn to accept yourself as well.

* * *

"IF . . . THEN . . ."

Similar to the idea behind drawing up our Plan of Action (see page 87), it can be helpful to try the "If . . . Then . . ." writing exercise. This specific journaling exercise is designed to prepare productive, healthy responses to uncomfortable, triggering scenarios or emotions like a craving: "*If* I feel X, *then* I will Y."

* ★ Set a timer for ten minutes.
* ★ Now write around dealing with an alcohol craving. For example: "*If* I feel lonely, *then* I will call a friend."
* ★ Keep writing until the buzzer goes.
* ★ Afterwards, read through what you've written. Could you action any of these suggestions in RL next time a craving comes on?

• •

GRATITUDE LIST

Expressing gratitude in any form can be beneficial to your health, but a great way to make it part of your everyday routine is by creating a gratitude list practice. There are a ton of "gratitude journals" available online that can give you prompts, or you can simply start by waking up each day and writing down three to five things you are grateful for in your life in a journal or notebook. Alternatively, you can do this before you go to bed to remind yourself of the good things you've experienced, which means you will go to sleep thinking of all the positives. Studies show that practising gratitude regularly can reduce stress levels, increase optimism and create new neural pathways.[2] Looking at the positives in your life can help you find perspective, especially during times when you are feeling depressed or unmotivated.

"I AM GRATEFUL FOR"

This next exercise plays into what you learned in chapter two about shifting your mindset to becoming more optimistic.

Over the next seven days, I want you to commit to writing down three things each day that you are grateful for in your life. To make this practice even more interesting, try to make your list broad and varied by including three new things each day – or by thinking of different aspects of the same topic.

I recommend using habit stacking by adding in this exercise to a daily routine you already have, like right after you brush your teeth in the morning or before you check your emails. James Clear, author of *Atomic Habits*, has created an easy-to-follow formula for habit stacking: "After/Before [CURRENT HABIT], I will [NEW HABIT]."

At the end of the seventh day I want you to reflect on how this exercise has changed your perspective and if you think it would be a helpful tool to add to your daily routine.

Monday

★ ....

★ ....

★ ....

Tuesday

★ ....

★ ....

★ ....

Wednesday

★ ....

★ ....

★ ....

Thursday

★ ....

★ ....

★ ....

Friday

★ ....

★ ....

★ ....

Saturday

★ ....

★ ....

★ ....

Sunday

★ ....

★ ....

★ ....

BULLET JOURNALING

Also known as a BuJo, bullet journaling is the ultimate means to stay organized, keep track of your mental health and set short- and long-term goals. You may have seen this kind of journal before, as it's a bit different from a traditional journal with lined pages. Instead, it contains pages full of small dots. This is done so you can both write and draw in it.

This is my favourite kind of journaling because it allows me to be creative outside of just writing and personalize the journal just for me. I like to use mine as an all-in-one, daily to-do list, habit tracker and traditional journal. Using the bullet points I can create graphs to track my weekly habits like movement, meditation and drinking enough water.

Filling in the little squares as I complete my tasks allows me to see my accomplishments on paper and gives me a tiny boost of dopamine, our reward chemical.[3] This can also be a great way to keep track of your alcohol-free days!

DREAM JOURNALING

Dream journaling is an interesting way to gain insights into your emotions and what's going on inside. When you stop drinking or seriously cut back, you may begin to have vivid dreams for a period of time. Even if they aren't "good" dreams, that's OK – dreams are an indication of deep sleep,[4] which is extremely important for your overall health, as this is when your body releases specific hormones that work to repair your muscles, bones, tissue and improve immune system functioning.[5]

Dream journaling is best done in the morning right after you've woken up, as this is when your dreams will be fresh in your mind. The idea is to write down whatever it is you remember even if it doesn't make sense. You can begin to look for patterns or recurring dreams and start to reflect on their meaning. Some of the world's greatest minds, such as Albert Einstein, Nikola Tesla and Mary Shelley, used dreaming to gain inspiration for their world-renowned ideas.

DREAM A LITTLE DREAM

After you have completed your "I am grateful for" exercise, choose a week to start dream journaling.

Before you go to sleep at night, place a pen and paper by your bedside. For seven days straight, when you wake up, write down anything you remember from your dreams. If you don't remember your dreams, write down how you feel and what current state of mind you are in. At the end of the week, reflect on what you've written. Are there any patterns or recurring dreams? What insights can you gain about how you are currently feeling from these dreams?

Monday   Tuesday

★   ★
....

★   ★
....

★   ★
....

Wednesday   Thursday

★   ★
....

★   ★
....

★   ★
....

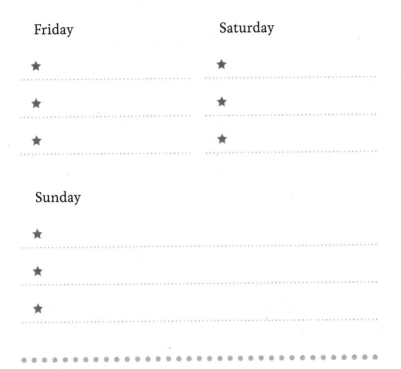

Friday

★
....

★
....

★
....

Saturday

★
....

★
....

★
....

Sunday

★
....

★
....

★
....

REFLECTION JOURNALING

The *Cambridge Dictionary* defines "reflection" as the activity of thinking about your own feelings and behaviour, and the reasons that may lie behind them. As you begin to gain further insight into yourself through your soberish journey, a reflection journal can be the perfect way to gain a deeper understanding of your past experiences and your current patterns of behaviour. It can also help you to find new perspectives. This type of journal is the perfect place in which to learn about your values and priorities and where you want to make changes in your life.

I have kept a reflection journal since my time in treatment, where I first learned the practice. At the end of each night, I would write down how the day went, if

I experienced any overwhelming emotions and if there was anything I needed to apologize to someone for (this could also include myself). While this approach fits into the tradition of the 12 Steps, I've continued to find this specific practice to be an extremely important way to keep myself honest, not hold on to resentments and to learn from any mistakes I may have made that day. Keeping a reflection journal can be a great tool for your own journey as it will allow you to face issues head on, rather than practise avoidance, as you may have done in the past by using alcohol as a distraction.

EVENING REFLECTIONS

You can find thousands of amazing reflections prompts for free online, but a great place to start is with the following practice.

Each night before bed, take ten minutes to write down and reflect on these questions:

* ★ Did I learn anything new about myself today?
* ★ Did I take time to practise my preventative rituals?
* ★ How did I deal with any uncomfortable emotions that came up?
* ★ Did I handle today's stressors to the best of my abilities?
* ★ Do I owe anyone an apology?
* ★ Am I happy with how today went? If not, what can I do to change the outcome or how I feel about it?

Monday

★
....

★
....

★
....

Tuesday

★
....

★
....

★
....

Wednesday

★
....

★
....

★
....

Thursday

★
....

★
....

★
....

Friday

★
....

★
....

★
....

Saturday

★
....

★
....

★
....

Sunday

★
....

★
....

★
....

START WRITING

So there you have it: there is no right or wrong way to journal. If you like the idea, you could commit to a daily practice as part of your POA, or just dive in whenever you are in the mood. And you can combine the different journaling techniques we've looked at in this chapter in whichever way suits you best – or maybe even make up your own.

Allow your journal to be as unique as you are, and it could be a friend for life along the path of your soberish journey. Soberish grapevine member Jess A. explains:

> *Journaling has been tremendously healing for me in my journey. Most of the time I don't know what to write, but once my pen hits the paper it starts flowing. I can honestly say revelations have come to me while writing in my journal. I do a lot of self-reflection with writing. Something about the connection between mind and pen, paper is beautiful. I write with no shame, no secrets, no judgement. I look back at my entries and sometimes cry with how much I have grown. It's an outlet that has helped me find out more about myself, and at times it has even been a spiritual experience.*

Journaling can be a great way to set yourself positive goals and to track your progress toward these as part of your POA. Besides being a way to hold yourself accountable, it can be a safe space in which to be creative and dream. You can even create your own journal for manifesting, a subject that we're going to be delving into next.

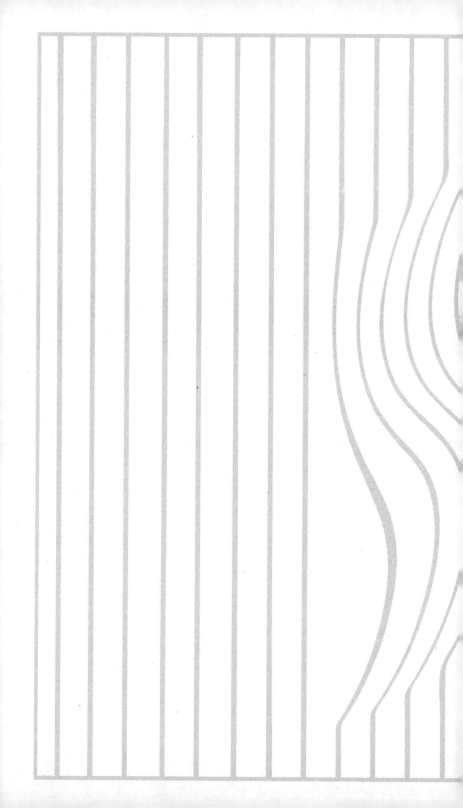

CHAPTER 13

Reclaim Your Power: Conscious Manifestation

Manifestation and its many practices are a huge part of my personal soberish toolkit. I truly believe that the companies I have built, the professional and personal successes I have had and the fruition of this book is all thanks to my manifestation practice. The best way to describe my idea of manifestation is "the attainment of intentions", as defined by Paul Hokemeyer, PhD, a clinical and consulting psychotherapist and author of *Fragile Power: Why Having Everything Is Never Enough*. To me, this means the practice of focusing and taking action toward whatever it is I want to manifest in my life.

A great example of how I practise manifestation in my life is through my vision boards. To some, these may just look like a collage of goals to aspire to, but to me these are foundational pieces on my journey toward bringing those desires to life. When I sit down to create these boards, I'm not only participating in a creative outlet, I am physically prioritizing what it is that I want to manifest into my life. Each photo or positive affirmation I glue onto my board is like a brick being laid over a concrete slab in my mind, solidifying my desire to obtain my goals.

I fill my vision boards with mindsets, mantras, job descriptions, retail images of things I'd like to purchase – you name it. I look at this board as a roadmap to my future, so that I can actually visualize what it is I want for my future in tangible form. When I'm done with each board, I add it to my wall in a place where I can look at it every day as a reminder of my goals and priorities. When I'm feeling unmotivated or am going through a rough patch, I can look at my board and remember that I'm in this for the long game – bad days pass but so do opportunities.

One of the reasons people often fail at following through with their resolutions of lifestyle habit changes is because they get excited in the moment, but forget about their vision over time. Without a vision there can be no goal. By having a vision board in your home, available for you to see every day, you can keep your priorities and goals in the forefront of your mind.

MANIFEST YOUR DESTINY

We looked at a version of a vision board back in chapter 3, when you created a booze board. However, a proper vision board is different, as it is all about what you *do* want to attract into your life, and instead of putting it away, you are going to display this piece where you will see it every day so that it primes your brain to recognize any opportunities that present themselves. Images imprint themselves on our minds more powerfully than words alone, and the more we look at the images (including images of words) on a vision board, the more likely we are to prioritize the things that they represent.[1]

You will need:
    any kind of large board to work on, e.g. a piece
       of poster board, a cork board or a pin board
    scissors, pins, double-sided tape and/or a glue-stick
    magazines, postcards and photos
    paper and pens
    markers, stickers, paint, glitter, dried flowers

★   First, make a list of your personal goals and priorities, which you'd like to manifest into your life over the next few months to year.

Write or print these out in large, colourful letters and cut them out.

★ Go through your magazines and photos, and cut out any images or pieces of text that represent your goals and priorities, and that make you happy when you look at them.

★ Stick your cut-out images and words onto your board. You can draw directly onto it too.

★ Add embellishments to make it fun! This is your board so put whatever you want on it that speaks to you. You can use stickers and scraps of fabric, seeds or dried petals. Take your time over it.

★ Once you have finished putting your board together, pin or tape it up in a place where you can look at it every day as a reminder of the things you'd like to attract into your life.

THE CORE PRINCIPLES OF MANIFESTATION

A vision board taps into the fact that our thoughts and beliefs about the world and ourselves shape our reality. As we saw in chapter 2, the downside to this is that it means cognitive distortions and hurtful comments from others can have detrimental effects on our overall wellbeing and self-image, even if they aren't true. But like everything else in life, there are two sides to this coin, and when we harness the power of positive thinking to shape our reality we can begin to attract what we desire. To manifest your priorities, life goals and dreams it's important to practise the following principles consciously.

HAVE A CLEAR VISION OF WHAT YOU DESIRE

Without a destination, the journey can seem aimless or take longer than expected. Imagine there's a new restaurant in town that you want to try, but you have no GPS, no map and no address for it. Now, you could drive around tirelessly in the hope of finding this place, but more than likely you'll be out of luck.

The same concept can be applied to your desires. With no GPS, no plan and no vision, accomplishing your goals is going to be like throwing darts at a board with a blindfold on. It's not impossible, but why make things harder for yourself when you can create your own map through manifestation? Setting goals and intentions through manifestation is like finding the restaurant address and using your GPS to get there. Once you have a clear direction in mind, the actions and behaviours you make will begin to align with your desires.

KNOW YOUR INTENTION

As with anything else you do in life, it is imperative to know your "why". *Why are you taking action? Why is this a priority to you? Why is this your goal?* When you know your intention behind your desire, you can put your time and energy into manifesting the desire into a reality. If the desire is inauthentic or doesn't align with your core values, you are less likely to put in the effort required to obtain your goals. But if your intentions are purposeful, you will feel compelled by your true values and priorities to take action.

As I look at my current vision board, I see many different photos, quotes and doodles that all symbolize the future I want to build for myself. A magazine clipping of a beautiful home, words that read "power, strength and routine", but most importantly in the middle of my board sits a piece of paper with a paragraph I wrote after a guided visualization at the 2019 MindBody Conference. During this guided visualization, the speaker asked us to look into our future. After the meditation had ended, the audience was asked to write down what we saw. This is what I wrote:

> *I saw my future. I am smiling. I had arrived. Accomplished. A mother. A wife. A boss. I am wearing a knotted blouse, skinny jeans and a pair of Louboutins. My hair is long and sits in a high ponytail. I am holding a little girl. He [my future husband] looks at me with adoration. I have everything I have ever wanted and I am giving back. I cannot wait to get there and to share this. I am her. This is what I am fighting for. What I deserve.*

This is the vision I hold of my future, and everything I do each day is a way to work harder toward that goal. If an opportunity arises that doesn't align with this vision, I pass on it. I ask myself daily, "Is this serving my higher purpose? My ultimate goals?" If the answer is no, then I don't do it. Everything I do is to live out my intentions.

"I AM . . ."

If you believe that you can't, then you can't. If you believe you are undeserving then the universe won't give you what you desire. More than likely, you haven't reached some of your goals because you have internalized the belief that you can't achieve them. You must throw this thinking out the window and tear off your rear-view mirror. That is about looking toward the past, and we are not going that way. From now on, I want you to adopt the mindset of "*I am*". Not even "*I'm going to be*", as this still implies doubt. You are now manifesting with certainty. Just like in my message to myself on my vision board, I speak in terms of "I am": "I am happy", "I am succeeding" . . . The energy and beliefs you put out into the universe are what you will receive, so start putting out that which you desire, that which you are.

PRACTISE ALIGNMENT

As with our Plan of Action (see page 97), in order to practise alignment we need to match our actions in parallel to our goals. If your goal is to change your relationship with alcohol, rather than just sitting about and wishing for change, start taking action to get closer to your goal. Examples in this scenario would be removing alcohol from your house, avoiding scenarios where alcohol is the central activity and finding a community that has the same values as you now do. Even if you're sober curious and unsure of what you want your relationship with alcohol to be, start acting the way you would in situations if you were a non-drinker. Observe yourself in these scenarios and ask which version of yourself is more aligned with your higher self, which is the wise, inner part of yourself that is free of ego and in tune with your true purpose.

TRUST THE PROCESS

This is probably the hardest principle, in my opinion, because it involves patience. You can set everything up, be as prepared as possible and you still may need to wait before your goals become a reality. Sometimes the timing isn't right, or you're not as prepared as you might think you are. Just remember that what is meant for you will find you. We live in a time when we crave instant gratification and we want everything now. We are used to getting next-day deliveries and being able to binge-watch entire series in one day. While quick is good for packages, it's not always the best for big lifestyle changes. You want to be fully prepared and ready for the opportunities you desire as they are presented to you. Being able to practice patience and acceptance is key to manifesting. Trust in the "*I am*" process and know you will have the outcome you want, you may just not know when.

TALKING ABOUT THE POWER OF MANIFESTING

Emma Mumford is an award-winning coach, mentor and leading Law of Attraction and manifestation expert. I caught up with her to ask her about the Law of Attraction and how manifesting works.

What is your personal definition of manifestation?
The Law of Attraction is one of the seven energetic laws of the universe; it's the notion that like attracts like and we are always creating our reality. Whatever you put out into the universe comes back to you, whether that's positive energy or negative energy. Think about it – I'm sure you've had a day where you've mentioned an annoyance to a friend or colleague, then something else happens and you voice it again, and then by the end of the day you feel like, "It's just been one of those days!" On the flip side, I'm sure we've all had those days too where something exciting has happened and we've told our loved ones about it. Then something else amazing happens and by the end of the day you feel like, "Wow, today was really my lucky day!" This

is the Law of Attraction in action. The Law of
Attraction is the law we work with to manifest
our dreams into reality through intention, whereas
manifestation is the physical manifestation of our
desire. There are no limits to what you can manifest –
you could manifest money, emotions, healing, a house,
relationships, your dream career and so much more!

How can an individual use manifestation to improve their mental health and overall wellbeing?

The Law of Attraction can really help you transform
every area of your life. Six years ago, I was anxious,
depressed, had an unhealthy relationship with alcohol
and had no idea how to love myself. Fast-forward to
now, and working with manifestation has helped me
to do the inner work, heal my limiting beliefs and
fears, learn how to love myself and live a positive
and happy sober life. Manifestation is really only the
beginning when you get onto your wellbeing or even
spiritual journey – you want to do and feel better,
which has a positive knock-on effect in all areas of
your life. It's also something that can be very easily
integrated into a morning practice to set you up
for manifesting and wellbeing success throughout
the day.

Can manifesting be useful to early sobriety? If so, how?

Absolutely! In my experience, I wouldn't focus on
setting an intention (goal) to be fully sober at first, as
that may feel like a big stretch for you in the beginning.
I would personally set intentions around feeling
happier or healing the belief or pattern within you
that creates an unhealthy relationship with alcohol.
It may not even be that deep; it could just be setting an
intention around not feeling socially pressured to drink
or even just feeling happier and more fulfilled within

yourself. The secret is to connect to the emotion you want to feel and work with your current emotions to release anything holding you back and to attract your desired outcome to you. Affirmations could be a great way to start this journey off for you.

What are some examples of manifestation exercises you can do at home?

There are lots of fantastic practices and rituals you can do each day to manifest abundance and your desires into your life. I would first of all recommend that you have a look at my Five steps to the Law of Attraction videos and content on my channels to help you better understand the process and what you need to do. From there, you can then try a few practices to determine what your manifesting superpower is and which ones feel good to you. I would recommend trying:

- ★ creating a vision board
- ★ scripting (writing down a few intentions for the next day)
- ★ journaling
- ★ visualizing your desires as if they've already happened
- ★ writing a goals list for the year ahead
- ★ manifestation meditations
- ★ daily intention-setting through your daily practice

If you'd like to find out more about these practices and how they work, I have videos for each of them on my YouTube channel.

What are some myths about manifesting? What is it versus what it isn't?

There are lots of myths and misconceptions when it comes to the Law of Attraction which I've come to realize over the last six years of my journey. The first is that I actually believe there are five steps in the manifestation process rather than the traditional three of ask, believe and receive. My five steps are:

* ask
* believe
* trust
* let go
* receive

Another myth I see often is an old-school teaching around fearful thoughts manifesting. This is such a damaging teaching because it installs fear so easily implies that you must always think positive thoughts! The reality is that, yes, our vibration (energy) does create our reality, but it's only our consistent vibration that does. We humans have around 80,000 thoughts a day; if every single one of them manifested, we'd live in a very chaotic universe, so it's very lucky they don't! Feeling is healing at the end of the day, and I'm a true believer in that what you resist persists, so by diving into the thought or feeling coming up you can effectively release this and raise your vibration, rather than suppressing it and feeling fearful still.

Anything else you feel is important to add?

One last thing I would add is that when taking your power back from alcohol, really look at your relationship with self-love and self-worth. Working on this will help you to form a healthy relationship with yourself where you can make more empowered decisions from an aligned space. A great affirmation I always work with and I'd recommend using is "I reclaim my power and call back all the lost pieces of myself". Each and every day, we give our power away both consciously and unconsciously, so repeating this mantra daily will be a powerful first step in reclaiming your power.

THE FUTURE YOU WANT IS MANIFESTING RIGHT NOW

Manifesting isn't the same thing as wishful thinking: it's about training your brain to focus on what you *do* want to attract into your life, rather than wasting precious energy and resources on worrying about what you don't. It's also about prioritizing your goals and aligning your actions with these, so that you are consciously and actively collaborating with the universe. As we've seen, you can manifest pretty much anything – from your ideal job, to what kind of drinking behaviours you want to adopt, to the people you want to surround yourself with – which brings us on to our final tool: community.

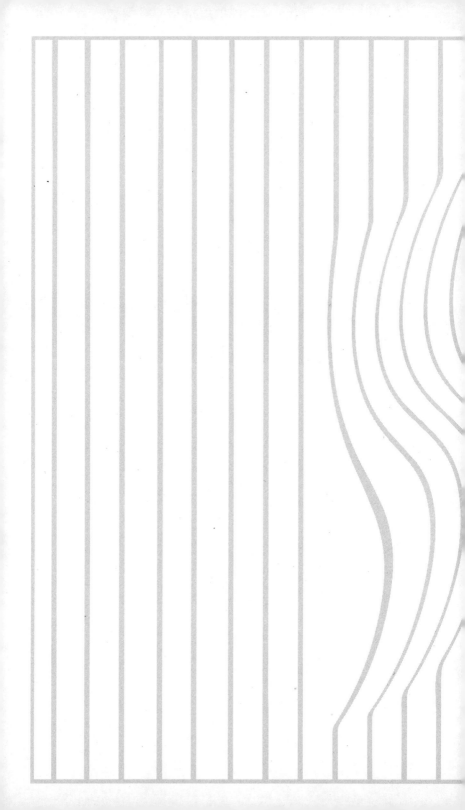

CHAPTER 14

Build a Community: Create Your Soberish Support System

The foundation of your entire toolkit is going to be your soberish support system. This can include loved ones, friends and other sober/ish/sober-curious people who support your journey and who you can lean on in tough times. Although the process itself of changing your relationship with alcohol is ultimately your path to walk alone, you will need people there to walk alongside you to remind you why you are doing this and love you when you can't love yourself.

PRACTISING THE ACCEPTANCE OF LOSS

Like the toolkit itself, each individual's support system will look different. Some of us may be blessed with families who support our choices around drinking by keeping alcohol out of the house if we live with them, or removing the focus from it in other ways if we don't. They may decide to drink less or not at all around us, and they may even be willing to participate in group therapy to tackle any wider issues connected with drinking for self-medication. However, while there are those who are blessed with caring people around them, the sad truth is that for some of us support on our soberish journey will not necessarily be found on the home front and we may even lose some friends along the way.

If you come from a family or a group of friends that drinks heavily, they may not understand your decision or be happy about it. It's important to remind yourself that this is in no way a reflection on you, it is a projection of their own relationship with alcohol. Changing your habits will make others around you question theirs, and if they also struggle with alcohol but aren't ready to face this truth, they're not going to like it. This relates to a concept known as "the shadow self", a term coined by psychoanalyst Carl Jung. The idea of the shadow self is the side of ourselves that we deem unacceptable or find shameful.[1]

You may find that if your family and friends remain unsupportive of your choices around alcohol, you may even need to separate yourself from them to avoid being in a toxic environment. It can be hard to accept the lack of support from certain people at first, but try to remember you were like them not long ago. How would you have reacted if someone close to you decided they were going to stop drinking while you were halfway through your first bottle of pinot? I know for a fact I would have felt personally attacked and asked myself the same questions those around us will ask themselves now, e.g.: "If Kayla isn't drinking anymore and we drink together all the time, does that mean I have a problem?" Instant defence mode.

If you're anything like me, I had a tendency to surround myself with others who drank the way I did so I could hide in plain sight. No one was questioning my drinking or my toxic behaviours as the big sister of a fraternity and my college best friend sure wasn't saying shit after I picked her up from jail after her third DUI (arrest for driving under the influence). We tend to flock to people who validate or enable our behaviour by acting in similar ways to ourselves, or by being "yes men/women". Becky isn't going to call you out at brunch for your fourth mimosa because she's finishing her third and Brad isn't going to pull you aside to ask if you're OK after watching you crush your six pack of Coors before halftime. People like this aren't real friends, they are drinking friends, and there is a huge difference.

Real, quality friends (who you *will* find on this journey) will call you out when you're doing something that is harmful to you. They will be concerned if you're not doing well and they will want the best for you.

The friends I have now let me know if they see me backsliding, they hold me accountable for my actions and they show up for me when I'm going through hard times. When I was going through my separation, every single woman in my "sober crew" showed up for me, emotionally supported me and didn't hesitate to pick up the phone when I called or swing by the house when I felt at risk of backsliding. However, when I was drinking, not once did any of my drinking buddies pull me aside to talk about my behaviour or ask if I was OK, regardless of the number of times I was hospitalized, arrested, screamed at them, got kicked out of bars or worse. If this is sounding all too familiar then it may be time to go friend shopping. The good news is that there is an amazing community of like-minded individuals out there, just waiting to support you — all you have to do is reach out.

BUILDING A NEW SYSTEM

So where does one find these incredible, unconditional new friends? The first place I always tell people to look is online. Social media platforms such as Instagram, Meta and Reddit have extremely strong and informative communities for the sober/ish/sober-curious. These range from pages dedicated to giving you resources, to large groups that offer support meetings, private group messaging and even coaching.

Every single person who I now consider a close friend, I met through what I call "sobergram". These are the same individuals I see regularly for brunch, movie nights or group walks. And the ones who don't live near me I text or FaceTime almost every day. There is just something so unique about the bonds you will make through this journey. You may even find in some instances that the connections are deeper and even more meaningful.

Personally, I never felt truly seen or like I actually fit in somewhere until I found this community. They are the reason I'm writing this book and the reason I'm able to be so resilient through difficult times. This is also why I created a community specifically for you, which already exists online and which is called "Join Soberish". I wanted to give you a place to start and build from. In this space you will find resources, information, inspiration and other people just like you searching for answers. We also hold weekly meetings where you can come and connect with others on their own soberish journeys, ask questions, share what you're going through or simply just listen and hold space for others. Why not include these in your own POA, as an ongoing source of emotional support?

PLACES TO START

Checking out communities online means that you don't have to commit to anything right away. There is no need to stand up in front of a bunch of strangers and tell your story until you feel ready.

★ **Instagram:** @joinsoberish – our personal soberish community. Using the hashtags #soberish, #sobercurious, #thedryclub, #soberlife, #sobercommunity, #mindfuldrinking and #californiasober you can find and connect with other like-minded individuals who are active in the space. I also recommend following your favourite quit-lit authors and thought leaders on this platform. You can find other similar accounts by going to the "following" list of @joinsoberish and following people that we follow.

* **Facebook/Meta:** Start by searching keywords like "sober curious" or "mindful drinking" and a list of private groups will appear. Top groups I would recommend are "Sober n Out for the Sober Curious", "Sober Sisters", "SoberMotivation", "On the Mocks" and "Break Free: A Community for the Sober and Sober Curious".

* **Reddit:** If you're looking for peer support, the Reddit community is great! I would recommend /r/stopdrinking: a support group in your pocket, and /r/sober: for getting sober and sober living.

* **In-person/online meetings**: The following groups are all programmes that I would recommend trying out to see where you best fit in:

    * **SMART Recovery**: an alternate, science-based support group.

    * **Refuge Recovery**: a Buddhist approach-based support group.

    * **Moderation Management**: a support group for those looking to manage their drinking through behaviour change.

    * **HAMS**: a peer-led group that provides support and information to those who want to change their drinking habits.

Soberish grapevine member Kate G. stopped drinking at the age of 24. She says:

Sober Instagram was a great way to meet other people who choose not to centre their life around drinking. For example, when I first stopped drinking, I was living in Seattle, so I would look through hashtags like #soberseattle and DM anyone that was also sober. I eventually formed a group message with some of these people from sober Instagram, and we would make plans for dinner, walks, coffee, etc.

There is a whole new soberish community out there. If you are shy, it may feel challenging to reach out to strangers, but I promise it will be worth it. Those strangers can soon become friends. And if you can't find a supportive community, you could create your own.

A WHOLE WORLD IS OUT THERE, WAITING

Joining a soberish community is one of the most powerful things you can do. Your soberish support system will be familiar with the sorts of experiences you have gone through, and will help to keep you motivated to look toward the future and avoid the sort of backsliding behaviours we are going to be looking at in chapter 15. They may even take part with you in some of the new tools that you have at your disposal, such as intuitive movement and meditation, manifesting or swapping recipes for delicious, nutritious meals. Online and in RL, you will find a new group of friends who don't need to drink to have a good time, and who will be there to cheer you every step of the way and listen to you when you hit a bad patch. Why not include socializing with them as part of your POA? And another great thing: wherever they live, these people will likely become real friends, which means that the energy flows both ways and you will be able to return the favour.

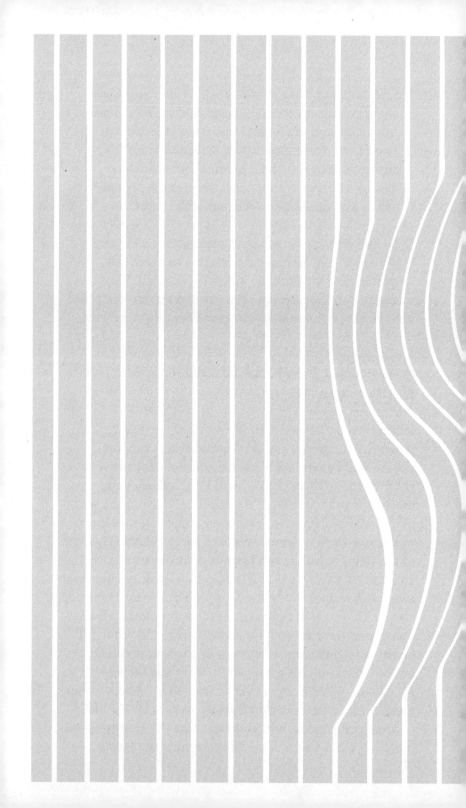

Putting Your Toolkit Into Action

PUTTING YOUR TOOLKIT INTO ACTION

You have your new tools at the ready, you're good to go . . . and then, life happens. Even when you are feeling confident and excited about discovering what being soberish could look like for you, things are rarely that easy. There may be times when your plans unravel, your intentions come undone and you find yourself backsliding toward old habits. That's why we are going to be examining the types of behaviour that can act as red flags at those moments. Self-awareness is key, right?

Once you realize that backsliding might be possible, you can do something about it. To help support your soberish forward progress, we're also going to be taking a look at the importance of maintaining your energy levels through proper self-care that incorporates the sorts of helpful practices that we looked at in Part Two. And finally, having identified some of the behaviours and attitudes that are no longer serving you earlier in this book, you're going to discover how to shed these and replace them with a new identity that reflects the highest version of yourself and which aligns with your true priorities, values and goals.

You are about to discover how giving
up booze isn't about denying yourself
anything – it's about gaining an incredible
life along with the resilience to cope with
anything that gets in the way of that.

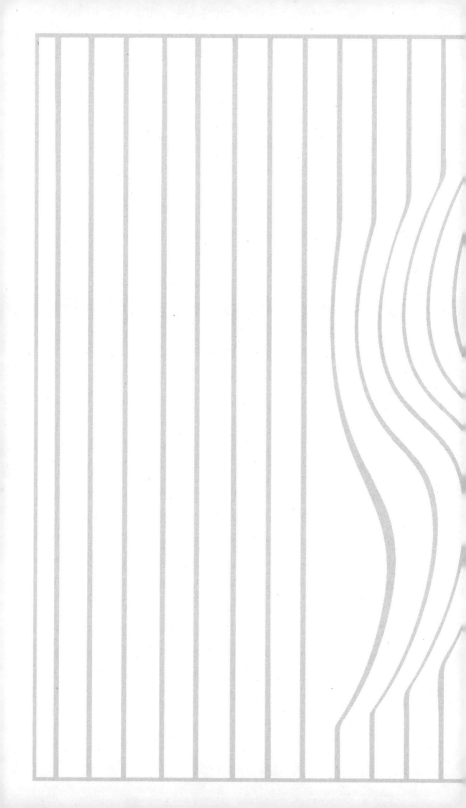

CHAPTER 15

Beating Backsliding Behaviours

Like so many others, my journey started as a sober-curious one. Before I was able to really commit to a new soberish lifestyle, I tried testing the waters and experimenting for weeks or even months at a time before I was ready to take long-term action. During this time, I had periods where I fell back into old drinking habits because I really didn't have a soberish foundation in place. I also didn't know how to string time together because I didn't know the signs of what I call "backsliding behaviours". Learning to identify these behaviours allowed me to take action before I took the first drink, which put me back in the driver's seat.

Just like the achievements of a professional athlete, your success on this journey will be an accumulation of hard work, practice, patience, learning from your mistakes and identifying potential problems before they happen. The better you are prepared for the general future, the less likely you will be to fall back into old habits. However, I've said it before and I'll say it again: this journey is *not* linear. Most of us will experience a backslide into old behaviours, more than once, before we get our baby soberish legs sturdy. We may even change some of our long-term goals around drinking during the course of our journey. The most important takeaway should be that you learn from your experience, show yourself compassion and allow a misstep to solidify your decision to change your relationship with alcohol. Do you think I just woke up one day after years of binge drinking and said to myself, "Yup, today is the day!" No. It was a conscious, difficult effort with a lot of ebbs and flows, but boy, was it worth it.

SIGNS OF BACKSLIDING BEHAVIOURS

Using your new self-awareness and tools that can help with this, like meditation, intuitive movement, somatic intuition and journaling, you can learn how to tune in to your emotions and become aware of the signs of "backsliding behaviours". These usually occur during the period before you actually take a drink (or drinks, for most of us). As we found out when we started to draw up our POA at the end of Part One, we all have warning signs, like red flashing lights screaming at us "Do Not Go This Way!" The trick is to remove the idea that "this time it will be different", because it won't, and actually listen to these warnings.

Let me break the signs of backsliding behaviours down into categories, so that you can better identify them.

ISOLATION

"Social isolation" happens when we cut ourselves off from others. This can look like not answering your phone, cancelling plans, not showing up to your support meetings and seeking time alone instead of connection. Isolation can be dangerous because it disconnects us from our sources of emotional support and creates loneliness.

I have a tendency to isolate myself when I'm overwhelmed or stressed, because it feels like a way of protecting myself. The last thing I want to do is answer a call or hit up a Zoom meeting to talk to people about what I'm feeling. But the problem with this defence mechanism is that it has a tendency to make our negative emotions like depression and anxiety worse.[1]

We can also experience emotional isolation as a result of social isolation. When this happens, it's as if we have shut down our emotions and stopped communicating them with others. Like social isolation, we may do this to protect ourselves from more distress.

Spending time alone isn't inherently bad, but if our intention behind isolation is to practise avoidance, then we have a problem. To avoid isolation it's important you stay connected with your support system and show up even when you don't feel like it. Don't feel like talking on the phone? Try texting. Maybe you've been crying and you don't want to participate in a meeting. That's OK; just sitting in and listening not only keeps you connected but allows you to share space for others, which will make you feel better. It can be helpful to schedule a specific time to touch base, as that way you won't feel overwhelmed or caught off-guard.

ROMANTICIZATION

To romanticize alcohol means to think about old behaviours and situations in an idealized or unrealistic way. You see the experience through rose-tinted glasses, which makes drinking seem better or more positive than it actually was.

Romanticization can happen when we listen to our old party music or watch television shows that make drinking seem glamorous or appealing. (Cough, cough, shows *Euphoria*, *Skins* and *Degrassi*!) It could even involve purchasing alcohol for a "special event" or upcoming dinner party when you realistically don't need to have it in the house yet.

I tend to romanticize alcohol most when I'm out with friends, which is the opposite of how I started. In the beginning of my journey, it was the more negative situations that made me feel like drinking, but I'm at a place now where I have to be more mindful in celebratory-type situations. It's easy for me to look at friends taking shots or drinking to excess and think of the good times I used to have doing the same thing. But the difference between me and them back then was *my intention*. I wasn't drinking to enjoy the moment, I was drinking to deal with social anxiety and I also had no "off" switch. Now when I'm in a situation, I learn to "play the tape forward" (see page 237), which refers to visualizing the situation if I do decide to drink. I take into consideration what would happen if I didn't drink, if I did and stuck to my limit, or if I over-drank. Doing this helps me make the decision that is right for me without being impulsive.

AVOIDANCE

No one's path to a healthier relationship with alcohol is perfect, but another sign you're falling back into old patterns could be when you begin to avoid your current soberish or cut-back plan all together; you stop keeping track of your drinks and attending meetings, and you are no longer doing your daily preventative tasks (aka using the tools we looked at in Part Two). You can be at higher risk of this happening during the holiday season or when you're traveling because it's harder to stick to your regular routine.

The trick to avoid falling off track is to plan ahead. If you know you're going to be going out of town or hosting people at your home, be sure to set aside time for yourself. This can look like setting reminders on your phone, signing up early for support meetings or scheduling a call with a friend who is supportive of your journey.

For me, I know something is up when I stop exercising and meditating, avoid showering, start sleeping in late and get behind on my to-do list. These are some of the tools I use to keep myself on track, so when I notice I'm becoming avoidant of these, I make an emergency therapy session immediately, call a friend or get myself to a support meeting. It helps me to schedule my fitness classes and support meetings ahead of time so that I can plan around them. I also remember to practise self-compassion if I am at risk of backsliding, instead of making the situation worse by shaming myself. Life happens and sometimes we get off track: what defines our journey isn't what we forget to do but how we pick ourselves back up and push on.

DIGRESSION

Digression is a pretty common defense mechanism. We often use defence mechanisms to cope with feelings of stress or anxiety. For most of us, these behaviours can be unconscious, so we don't even know we're doing it. When it comes to drinking specifically, you may find yourself spending time with old drinking buddies or people who don't necessarily support your desire to stop or drink less. You may also start going out more often to bars, concerts, parties or other places that can trigger your desire to drink.

Again, what you really want to concentrate on is your *intention* behind these actions. Plenty of people feel comfortable jumping back into social situations |and hanging out with "drinking friends" in the beginning of their journey. If you feel confident and those around you support your decision then there's nothing wrong with living your best life. The risk lies in hanging around people who may keep offering you drinks even after you've declined, and those who don't support your new journey and may try to shame you into drinking with comments like "your drinking wasn't that bad" or "you're no fun if you just have one". People like this are not your real friends; frankly, they are energy vampires who lack insight and awareness around your interpersonal decisions. People like this will suck out your social and emotional energy, leaving you at higher risk for the "fuck-its". I noticed quite quickly that not drinking gave me much less patience for these kinds of people, wild parties and late nights. I had to learn how to navigate what I actually enjoyed spending my time doing and how to identify when my social battery was running low.

ANXIETY

When you stop doing your preventative behaviours (aka using the tools in your toolkit) or get out of your normal routine, anxiety can set in. Perhaps your work environment has become more stressful recently or you went through a painful breakup. If your anxiety and stress levels are up, and your sleep hygiene and preventive behaviours are down, you are more prone to seek out alcohol to deal with the discomfort.

This was basically my entire 2022 experience: chronic anxiety. I explained earlier how I went through a painful breakup and ended up living with my parents, quitting a job at a company I helped build from the ground up and then writing this book. I can honestly say that for me this year has been almost, if not just as anxiety-provoking as trying to quit drinking. The difference has been sticking to my POA and focusing on my goals even when every cell in my brain was yelling at me to stay in bed and give up. Committing to my fitness classes, therapy sessions, meditation practice and showing up to support groups kept me from completely falling off the rails. Reminding myself that I was playing the long game helped too. Because even if present-day Kayla didn't want to do it, Kayla in six weeks' time would be grateful I did, so I carried on.

DEPRESSION

Similar to isolation, depression involves feelings of sadness or loneliness that won't go away and which can trigger a backslide into drinking. Signs you are feeling depressed can look like cancelling important appointments such as therapy, no longer practising intuitive movement, avoiding your self-care routines and sleeping a lot.

However, it's important to note there is a difference between feeling depressed and having clinical depression. Clinical depression requires a diagnosis and is characterized as a more severe form of depression, whereas situational depression is usually short-term.[2] Situational depression is usually triggered when we experience a significant change in our life – and I would say going soberish could involve a considerable adjustment. Creating lifestyle changes can help you reduce the symptoms of situational depression while you get over the hump of the early days of your soberish journey. Many of these changes can be found in your soberish toolkit: regular movement, eating a well-balanced diet, practising proper sleep hygiene or hopping into a support group.

Now that we've identified some of the warning signs that we are at risk of backsliding into our old drinking ways, what to do about them? We can start by managing our Body Battery.

CHARGING OUR BODY BATTERY

Many people who don't understand the concept of alcohol use disorder believe that it all comes down to a lack of "willpower" in the individual who is suffering, but that couldn't be farther from the truth.

I had the pleasure of being able to sit down with my good friend the therapist and sober coach Beth Bowen and get the full scope of her physiological concept of the "Body Battery", which explains how we are able to manage our mental, physical and emotional energy in order to give our brain enough space to function at its highest capacity.

According to Beth's Body Battery concept, your ability to make intentional decisions requires a healthy, high-functioning prefrontal cortex (PFC). The PFC is our "higher thinking" brain, which is responsible for our decision-making, impulse control and our personality, among other vital functions. When we misuse or overconsume alcohol, our PFC becomes compromised – resulting in the sort of brain damage we spoke about in chapter 1. When this happens, we can begin to act out of character because we are no longer behaving from a place of conscious, intentional decision-making. We may start to become more impulsive and participate in high-risk behaviours that we normally wouldn't do, or lose sight of our true priorities.

The Body Battery also "involves our limbic system, or our more 'animalistic' brain", as Beth explains it. She says, "The limbic system is composed of several smaller structures in our brain related to memory, processing emotions and, importantly, our survival instincts. To oversimplify it: the limbic system is interested in sex, drugs, and rock and roll . . . and it wants it NOW!" These two brain structures are constantly sending us opposite messaging. The prefrontal cortex is like the responsible friend who tells the limbic system to take it easy, while the limbic system is the wild friend who craves instant gratification. This is where awareness and understanding of the Body Battery comes into play. "Whichever brain structure is driving your brain bus is deeply dependent on the totality of your mental, physical and emotional energy at any given moment," explains Beth. This is why it is so important to learn how to manage and regulate the Body Battery, so that you can ultimately control who ends up in your brain's driver's seat.

THE BODY BATTERY CYCLE

Remember the drinking cycle we went over in chapter 1? The one we can't seem to break even after we promise ourselves and others we will never drink again? This is due to the impairment we have caused in our brain by alcohol misuse and is directly correlated to our Body Battery. The Body Battery can be thought of as the total sum of three different energies:

- ★ **Mental energy:** This is the energy you expend by thinking. Mental energy plays a part in your decision-making, memory and managing your emotions. You expend this energy when working through problems in your mind, learning something new, or when remembering something from the past.
- ★ **Physical energy:** This is the more general understanding of energy. It's about how your physical body exerts or gains energy through movement, rest, and proper nutrition. When you exercise, you exert physical energy to get stronger, release endorphins and build endurance.
- ★ **Emotional energy:** This is the energy you source from your emotions. Your emotional states have the power to boost or drain your emotional energy. An example of a "high energy boost" would come from a positive emotion

such as love or happiness, where a "high energy drain" would come from grief or rage.

These three types of energies combine to make up the Body Battery. To get a better visual, you can think of yourself as a smartphone that needs to be charged based on the scale of 0 per cent to 100 per cent charged. "Everything we experience throughout our day results in energy *burn* or energy *charge*," says Beth. "Every action, thought or emotion we experience throughout the day starts to chip away at our Body Battery. Alternatively, there are things we can do to juice up our Body Battery, too."

Examples of burning energy could include making a simple decision about what to eat for breakfast, which would drain your mental energy, or something more heated like getting into a row with your partner, which would consume 5 per cent of your emotional energy. On the flip side, you could take action to recharge your Body Battery by having a power nap, for example, which would boost your physical energy, or increasing emotional energy by participating in a hobby or activity that you're passionate about. (For me, this could be vision boarding or serving the online soberish community.)

Just like a real smartphone, the lower your Body Battery goes, the higher you are at risk of backsliding behaviours. This is because our limbic system (aka Mr Instant Gratification) starts to slip into the driver's seat, which makes us more likely to act out of impulse or the desire to feel good. "This is why your resolve not to drink can wane so dramatically by 5pm," explains Beth. "Your prefrontal cortex is no longer driving the bus because your energy is so drained."

LEARNING TO CHARGE AND RESTORE THE BODY BATTERY

Now that you have awareness of the Body Battery, and how it works, here are a few tips on how to begin to manage your expenditure:

* **Practise essentialism:** Identify all of the decisions you need to make throughout your day and prioritize them: for example, *what needs to be done today, what can be done this week and what tasks can be given to others?* This can significantly help reduce the risk of decision-fatigue or feeling overwhelmed.
* **Remember that all emotions utilize energy:** Understand that no matter the emotion being utilized, you run the risk of burning through your Body Battery. Make sure to set aside time to restore and recharge yourself daily through having some downtime and using one of your soberish tools as part of your POA.
* **Enjoy intuitive movement:** Understand which physical activities *burn* your physical energy, and which ones *increase* it. Exercise is a great example. The majority of the time, intuitive movement increases our physical energy because it provides us with both physical and mental benefits like the release of dopamine and endorphins. Other times, if we are feeling tired out, or in need of rest but decide to exercise anyways, we can burn our physical energy and lower our Body Battery.
* **Practise "plugging in":** Regularly practise activities that create rest and capacity, like sleep, connection with loved ones, and mindfulness.

In my conversation with her, Beth Bowen stresses just how important a role our Body Battery can play in the way that our soberish journey unfolds:

> *The truth is this: willpower, in the choice to "drink responsibly" (or moderately, or not at all) is a mere fraction of the equation. A much larger part of our ability to make informed decisions around drinking requires a well-tended Body Battery, leaving us with capacity and a healthy balance of mental, physical, and emotional energy. When we're able to operate from our prefrontal cortex, we're much more likely to be able to align our intent with our actions.*

Resetting your relationship with booze isn't just a case of gritting your teeth and summoning up the willpower; it's about being genuinely kind to ourselves by learning to listen to our bodies and what they need. After all, the better we look after our Body Battery by managing our energy levels, the more chance we stand of avoiding backsliding behaviours and to keep making forward progress.

PLAY THE TAPE FORWARD

When it comes to redefining our long-term relationship with alcohol, an oldie but a goodie is the concept of "playing the tape forward". It's another way of saying "visualize what will happen if you do decide to drink". It's a great technique to use when you're in the middle of a craving or feeling triggered by an uncomfortable emotion. I used it a lot when I first stopped drinking, especially when romanticization kicked in and the little wine witch in my head would whisper in my ear, "*Just one won't hurt.*" Reminding myself that nine out of ten times my drinking ended with some sort of altercation, blacking out, or a hospital visit would swiftly shut up that little witch and lock her back in the attic where she belonged.

Playing the tape forward is a simple and effective mindfulness tool you can use at any time, because the only thing it requires is your mind. It does take practice, though – like any mindfulness technique you have to build it up like a physical muscle, but it's worth it. As soberish grapevine member Ashley M. puts it:

When I feel a craving coming on, particularly when it's at an inconvenient time like if I have work the next day, I like to play the tape forward in order to remind myself why I'm better off not drinking. I do things like think about the hangover I'd have the next day, and I recall the last time I had to work hungover and how miserable it was. This really helps because it often feels like no big deal to have a drink, but once you've had a few, there are so many consequences that can come your way.

HOW TO PLAY THE TAPE FORWARD

A great way to create a foundation for this practice is by setting aside five minutes every morning to play the tape forward, imagining both the negative and positive versions. You can incorporate this activity into your POA, as part of step five.

★ Envision the potential short- and long-term consequences of going off course, like a fight with your partner, being late for work, having a horrible hangover or, worse, getting a DUI, being fired or potentially hurting yourself.

★ Then rewind and replay the tape, only this time imagine your day if you stay alcohol-free or within the limit you've set yourself. What are some of the potential benefits of staying on track? Perhaps your work or school performance improves, you get better sleep, your skin starts to look refreshed or you get to spend more quality time with your family?

★ Having both visualizations at the forefront of your mind will help you reach for them quicker if you find yourself in a craving or being triggered.

LEARN PROPER SELF-CARE

Once you feel solid in identifying the behaviours described on pages 225–30, which indicate you could be at risk of backsliding, and are aware of how your Body Battery affects your choices and are on the way to mastering the "Play the Tape Forward" technique, you can turn your attention to focusing on preventing future backslides. To do, so you will need to create a healthy, sustainable self-care routine and put it into action.

First, let's get something straight first: self-care is not synonymous with being selfish, self-indulgent or spending money. Self-care is a whole-person approach to keeping yourself healthy, happy and on track to the highest version of yourself. Face masks, bubble baths and snacking on tubs of ice cream are all great, but I want you to go deeper, because at the end of the day a sheet mask is not going to stop you from picking up that bottle of wine – but real coping mechanisms will. According to Dr Matthew Glowiak of Southern New Hampshire University, "engaging in a self-care routine has been clinically proven to reduce or eliminate anxiety and depression, reduce stress, improve concentration, minimize frustration and anger, increase happiness, improve energy, and more."[3]

Self-care can also help you to relieve the pressures of everyday life that normally lead you to drink. Similar to the "Signs of Backsliding Behaviours" that we looked at earlier in this chapter, we can break down the areas of self-care into five core categories. Each category focuses specifically on an area you may need to be tending to a bit more than you probably do at the moment. In order for you to maintain your own happiness and sense of wellbeing, each of these areas of self-care should be present in your regular routine.

EMOTIONAL SELF-CARE

When you focus on emotional self-care, you are practising nurturing your inner feelings and emotions. This is probably something new to you – it was for me – so be gentle and patient with yourself. The beginning of your journey may bring up uncomfortable emotions, but processing and nurturing them can help you decrease your stress levels and calm your central nervous system (CNS). I know that self-compassion and care can be really hard when we are harbouring feelings of guilt or shame, but you are not alone in this journey and I promise that as time passes, so will these feelings. As you strengthen this practice over time, it will allow you to be better able to regulate yourself emotionally and improve your self-control, areas that may have been compromised in the brains of some of us due to our alcohol misuse. Again, this is why we stay away from the blame game. When brain chemistry is compromised, people act out of character. Practising positive self-affirmations around this can help you move forward, such as: "I am worthy of forgiveness," "I am working hard to be the best version of myself," "I am transforming into the person I want to be." You can look inside your soberish toolkit to practise emotional self-care by using mindfulness meditation (see chapter 10), staying connected to your support group (see chapter 14) and moving your body intuitively (see chapter 7).

TELL SOMEONE YOU ARE GRATEFUL

We looked at creating gratitude journals in chapter 12, but you can practise emotional self-care in any given situation by using gratitude to shift your perspective. According to Robert Emmons, the world's leading scientific expert on gratitude, gratitude is "an affirmation of goodness. We affirm that there are good things in the world, gifts and benefits we've received."[4] Expressing gratitude to others can help us to decrease our stress levels and improve our general mood.[5]

- ★ Today, think of three people that you are grateful to. These could be individuals who are in your life now, like family members or friends, or people who have been there for you in some way in the past, like a supportive teacher, mentor or former boss.
- ★ Over the next month, make a conscious effort to reach out and show them that you appreciate them. This could be by simply

giving them a compliment, sending them a
message of thanks or going out of your way
to do something kind for them.

★ Try to do this without any expectation of
acknowledgement or reward.

★ Afterwards, think about how showing your
gratitude made you feel, and whether it is
helping to change your relationship with
yourself as well as the other person.

PSYCHOLOGICAL SELF-CARE

When we practise psychological self-care we are
learning, thinking or growing. We do this so that we
can develop intrapersonally – i.e. within ourselves.
Some examples of this can involve challenging our
negative thinking, journaling, practising positive self-
talk, or disengaging with social media. As humans,
we have a natural inclination to think and focus on
the challenges in our lives, which is called "negativity
bias". Having this bias can lead us to focus more on the
negative emotions and events in our life, which can
make them seem more prevalent than they really are.
We want to nip this in the bud early on, and we can
start by reminding ourselves that a lot of the negativity
or discomfort we are feeling is coming from the
dysregulation our brain and body is going through
from alcohol misuse.

I personally find it helpful to take time away
from social media platforms in the same way that
others practise dry months or challenges. It's hard
not to get caught up in other people's highlight
reels and comparisons with them quickly lead me

down a slippery slope of depression and feelings of worthlessness. While certain platforms can be a great way to connect with the soberish community, research shows us that there is a direct link between the presence of social media and increases in anxiety and depression.[6] Writing out how you feel in a journal is another great way to destress and regulate your emotional experiences.

TURN OFF THE FEEDS

How much time do you spend online, scrolling through timelines? And how does this affect your mood? Here's a mini challenge for you: Commit to a social media-free month to improve your mental wellbeing.

Check off this activity once you have completed the month, and reflect on how you felt before and after this challenge.

PHYSICAL SELF-CARE

As I mentioned before, movement is one of the most fundamental and simple ways you can practise self-care. In our soberish toolkit, we went over intuitive movement, nutrition and the importance of good sleep hygiene. However, physical self-care can be as basic as brushing your teeth, drinking enough water or putting on clean clothes. These can seem obvious enough but when we're in an emotional rut sometimes we just don't have the energy.

At the beginning of my soberish journey I wouldn't shower or brush my teeth some days, not because I wanted to be unhygienic but because my sole priority was making it through the day without drinking. Just getting out of bed was difficult, let alone going for a run or a spin class. So if you are in that place just know you are doing nothing wrong – the only thing you need to think about right now is this journey. Hang in there.

Starting with the basics helped me build up to a solid exercise routine and eventually a healthy intuitive movement practice, so just keep taking those baby steps. Also try to get some proper rest and recharge your Body Battery.

PROFESSIONAL SELF-CARE

If you are a working professional like myself, it's important to have a healthy work–life balance. The key to professional self-care is learning how to set and stick to your boundaries. I cannot stress this enough and it's honestly something I struggle with myself to this day. I recently left a job that had no boundaries. While part of the problem was a toxic environment, the other part was my inability to say no to taking on more.

It's perfectly acceptable to be passionate about your career but when it bleeds into your personal life or is causing you burnout, like it did me, then, Houston, we have a problem! If this sounds like you, I get it. You want to make people happy and show up for your company. But the truth is simple: you can't pour from an empty cup. Trust me, I have tried – it only leads to burnout. According to the World Health Organization (WHO), burnout happens when you do not successfully manage your workplace stress, leading to feelings of energy depletion, exhaustion and increased mental distance from your job. It may also lead you to feelings

of cynicism for your job and those you work with.[7]
All of these negative emotions put you at greater risk
of backsliding or harming your mental health.

To avoid burnout, and generally have a better work–
life balance, you can begin with small changes. I started
by putting away my work laptop on the weekends
and muting my Slack notifications after 7pm so that
I wouldn't be tempted to check them. I also had a
conversation with my management and my team
about when I would be signing off for the day so they
understood that anything sent after 7pm wouldn't be
attended to until the next morning. Having these set
boundaries allowed for me to truly relax during the
evening and not be constantly checking my phone,
which in turn helped my relationship.

I didn't even realize until after I'd set firm
boundaries how much the imbalance of my work life
had negatively impacted my relationship or mental
health, which took time to mend. Thankfully, making
changes and taking action improved my wellbeing and
my relationship. It's important to remember your job
can impact those around you too if you do not have
a healthy work–life balance. It can be difficult to set
these boundaries at first, so try to give yourself small
rewards for sticking to them.

SWITCH OFF

Whether you work from home or go into an office,
establish clear end points to your work day. Having
a hard stop will help you to differentiate your work
time from your personal time, allowing you to be more

present at home. Having a hard-stop will also push you to be more organized with your schedule.

- ★ If you need to, set a reminder or an alarm on your phone or computer for when you plan to clock out at the end of the day.
- ★ Keep a calendar or a list of your weekly to-dos. I find it helpful to schedule my week ahead of time, as well as pencil in extra space in case something unexpected pops up.
- ★ Clearly outline your tasks, which will help you prioritize them. Break them up into smaller projects that you can do throughout the day or week.
- ★ Most importantly, evaluate your workload and remember that "No!" is a complete sentence. You are not obligated to fulfil tasks outside of your job description and although turning down projects can be difficult if you're a "company" man or woman, you will quickly find you can better execute what is already on your plate when you are not overwhelmed.

SPIRITUAL SELF-CARE

Spirituality can have many different meanings, but your concept can be whatever resonates best with you. Spiritual self-care does not have to involve religion (unless you want it to); it's about developing a deeper sense of meaning and understanding of yourself and the world around you. Research shows that those who have a concept of spirituality are more satisfied with their lives, have greater perceived social support, higher resilience to stress, and lower levels of anxiety than those who have no spiritual practice.[8] Similar to psychological self-care, this is about focusing on inner development and a connection to the highest version of yourself.

If you struggle with the concept of spirituality, that's perfectly fine. In the beginning of my journey I didn't have a real sense of spirituality or what it meant to me. I had grown up in organized religion but wasn't interested in practising as an adult. I tried to connect with a higher power when I was in 12 Steps as suggested but I've mentioned earlier how it felt inauthentic to me. I remember at one point I found myself talking to "Sky Daddy" in the sauna and I literally felt like I was failing some sort of test because no one was talking back and I wasn't getting any "signs". It felt like, "I'm literally talking to myself – *what am I doing.*" But I knew it was important to have a concept of a deeper meaning in order for me to feel grounded and have purpose, so I started with something that made sense to me: the universe.

Having a concept of something larger than myself at work gave me motivation to put out positive energy and project what I wanted to receive. And creating a connection to my version of the universe allowed me to access new parts of myself and find purpose in all of my life events. By practising spiritual self-care, I have been able to find more clarity in overwhelming situations, build resilience through hard times and experience more inner peace. Having a meditation and yoga practice has been extremely beneficial to my spiritual self-care, as has connecting with others in the soberish community.

YOU'RE ON YOUR WAY . . .

You are equipped with your toolkit and POA; you know the tell-tale signs of backsliding behaviours; you are aware of how important it is to look after your Body Battery and you know how to "play it forward" to imagine the outcomes of drinking versus not drinking. You understand the importance of self-care and the many different and equally important forms that this can take. You are on the verge of shedding your old ways and emerging as someone new, someone who is no longer defined by harmful habits and cravings. Now you just have to start living your best soberish life for real . . .

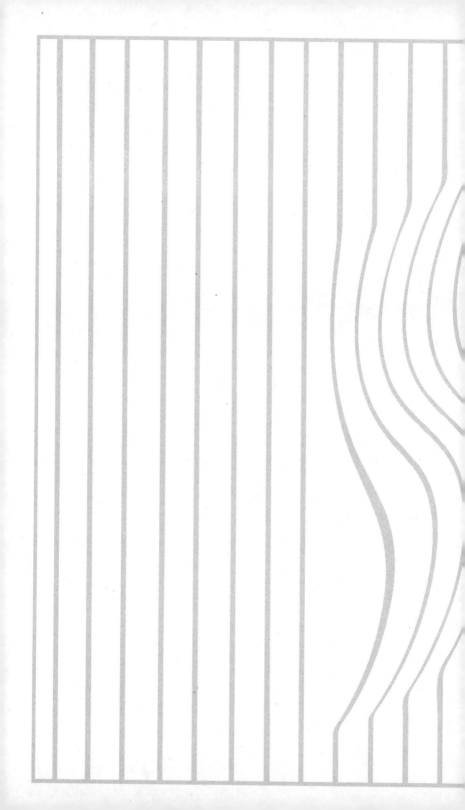

CHAPTER 16

New Me, Who Dis?: Recreating Our Self-Identity

So far, you have done a *ton* of introspection, re-evaluating your current lifestyle and choosing to take action to improve your relationship with alcohol.

I want you to take a moment for you to pat yourself on the back and give yourself credit for putting in the hard work. Many people wander through life and just accept things the way they are, or learn to live in discomfort – but not you. You've taken a leap of faith by going against the grain and prioritizing yourself, regardless of societal pressures. You are a disrupter. You are amazing.

Moving forward, I'm going to be helping you construct a new identity that reflects the highest version of yourself, one that aligns with your new values and priorities. If you're worried about making drastic overnight changes, don't be – this is a marathon, not a sprint. Together, we will be recreating your self-identity at a pace that works best for you. Get excited, as this is not just a new chapter in this book but a new chapter in your life.

Time is on your side. While some days or weeks may seem long, and progress may appear slow, remind yourself that any amount of progress is good progress. In fact, the more meticulous and focused you are on making these lifestyle changes, the more likely they are to stick. We tend to rush into things hoping for quick results – fad diets, over-exercising, giving up alcohol, sugar and carbs all at the same time – and then we wonder why we fail. It's because commitment is about more than just participation, it's about discipline and the long game. True commitment means we do something even if we don't feel like it, like waking up early for a run or finishing a paper that's due for class. While these activities aren't always the most enjoyable, they set us up for long-term success.

One of the personality characteristics I've noticed that seems to be popular among those of us who can't seem to make a new habit stick is that we have the desire but not the discipline. When it comes down to it, we will take the instant gratification of a nap over finishing our homework, of sleeping in instead of waking up for our run, or of drinking instead of sitting through those uncomfortable emotions. Adding discipline to your list of future values will help you tremendously when it comes to a lifestyle change.

Before I changed my relationship with alcohol I had zero self-discipline. I very much lived in the moment and my days were run by how well or hungover I felt from the night before. Alcohol was in the driver's seat of my life. Commitments to work shifts, classes, gatherings with friends all went out the window because my number-one priority was alcohol. Shifting my priorities and values to things that would serve me in the long term and help me to achieve my goals was a major shift in solidifying a soberish foundation for my life.

Again, the beautiful thing about our personal values and the way we show up for ourselves and others is that they are totally plastic. We can choose to make a change at any time, it comes down to our innate desire to truly make changes to improve our lives. Here are some questions to consider, moving forward:

★ How did/does alcohol impact my personality and character?
★ How centric was/is alcohol to my personal identity?
★ What parts of my personality may be affected by my relationship change with alcohol?

★ Who do I want to be without alcohol as a central role player in forming part of my self-identity?

★ What are my fears around changing my self-identity?

The last question – "What are my fears around changing my self-identity?" – was a big hurdle for me. From the time I started drinking at age 15, I had hitched my self-identity to alcohol as the wild-child party girl. As someone who suffered from low confidence and who lacked a strong self-identity, I craved connection and attention, and when I realized I could get a false sense of that through drinking and being the go-to girl for underage shenanigans, I latched on to the persona. This version of myself was constantly getting me into trouble, hanging out with the wrong crowd and putting me into dangerous situations – but I didn't care. I believed I had "friends" and people who needed me. And when you're young those things are top priority.

Even when I went away to university, I felt a strong need to continue to be the self-proclaimed party girl, being the big sister of a fraternity, making friends with the bouncers to get myself into the bars underage and drinking myself into oblivion to prove I was "that girl". It sounds so asinine now at age 30, but back then I felt like this was my life's purpose, which is why it was so hard to let go of that version of myself even when I recognized how problematic it was.

I probably spent years knowing I had an issue but the fear of creating a new version of myself was a big part of what held me back. If I only knew then what I knew now I could have made things so much easier for myself, but I've never been known to do things the easy way. I kept this persona going through uni until

I had finally exhausted myself and gotten into enough trouble to land myself in court-mandated rehab. While that wasn't where I stopped drinking, getting to meet other sober individuals while at treatment and meeting "cool girls" who didn't drink planted a seed for me, as I explained at the start of this book. Eventually, I decided my run was over and decided to retire my party girl persona. It was far from easy, but it was doable. And if I can do it, so can you.

IDENTITY FLUIDITY: SEASONS CHANGE AND SO CAN YOU

While we may not identify as "alcoholic" or even someone with an AUD, you may be surprised to find how deeply ingrained alcohol can be in our existing identity without us even knowing it. When I first changed my relationship with alcohol, I was shocked at how much of my life and my social activities centred on drinking. From girls' nights out, to football games, work dinners and even at wellness-related retreats focusing on mindfulness, alcohol was everywhere. Now, part of this was because I had been surrounding myself with other people who drank the way I did, but it made me curious as to what else was out there beyond the world of booze. *Could I really have fun and enjoy life as a young person sans booze?* Thankfully the answer was: *YES!*

Consider this – perhaps a regular week for you involves winding down with a cocktail in the evening while reading a good book, catching a bottomless brunch with friends on Sundays or going out to a party with them? None of these activities *require* drinking, yet we have just paired them together through societal pressure and the normalization of alcohol as a way to unwind or connect with others. I learned that I could participate in all the same activities that I had previously, only without drinking; I just needed to get past the initial social anxiety I was experiencing and the fear that everyone would judge me for not drinking.

To my surprise, in all the years I have been on my journey, I have run into less than a handful of negative experiences in which people have tried to peer-pressure me or shame me for choosing to prioritize myself over following the herd. This fear of others judging me or fixating on my drinking is actually the result of the "spotlight effect". According to psychological studies, the spotlight effect is a phenomenon whereby we tend to overestimate how much others notice aspects of our behaviour.[1] Let's say you walk into a party and instead of your usual drink of choice you have a non-alcoholic beer in your hand or a red Solo cup with seltzer water in it. Our anxious brain likes to try to convince us that everyone is hyper-focused on what we are doing and will bombard us with questions about our lifestyle change – when in reality no one cares. I say this in the kindest way possible, because others are too busy being worried about how they look or how they are behaving to notice what you are doing.

A great way to think about this is when you wake up with a blemish on your face and you instantaneously feel mortified: "Everyone is going to notice this, I look ugly, I most definitely cannot attend the party with *this* on my face!" Granted, these may be extreme thoughts, but they are ones that pop into my mind nonetheless. Then I try to remind myself when the last time I noticed someone's blemish was, or whether I can even recall what my roommate was wearing the day before. The answer is usually no, because again, I am too fixated on my own behaviour or appearance to worry about whether my roommate has a pimple or decided to re-wear her leggings. To sum it up simply – *no one cares* – and this is awesome news. Especially if you tend to suffer from social anxiety.

So how can you begin to build a layout for this higher version of yourself you want to become? Start small. Consider your current priorities, values and goals and how they align (or don't) with the person you want to become. It can be helpful to create a list or vision board of how you currently see yourself, and then create a separate one that represents the new version of you, similar to the way you did a vision board around what alcohol represents to you at the start of this book. Let's help you set a foundation for this with our next activity.

. . . .

REAPPRAISING YOUR PRIORITIES, VALUES AND GOALS

This is about creating a kind of blueprint for the person that you want to become during the course of your soberish journey. It involves taking a close look at your priorities, values and goals, and how they may be changing.

On a piece of paper write down the priorities, values and goals you have had over the last year before you made the decision to change your relationship with alcohol. Make this list as radically honest as possible; there is no judgement here. Remember you're already on the path to making better life decisions and your past decisions are what actually set you up to be where you are today. Here are some definitions and tips to help you get started with your lists:

Priorities: Our priorities may not be set in stone but tend to be the things that matter to us most in the present moment. In the past, my priorities were a bit skewed. When I was drinking heavily, I prioritized parties, social gatherings involving alcohol, and friends who enabled my bad habits, instead of prioritizing my mental health, my school work and my loved ones. What did your priorities look like before coming across this book? And what do you want them to look like moving forward as we bring you closer to your higher self? Here are some examples of healthy priorities that I try to focus on in my own personal life; feel free to check-mark or highlight any priorities that align with your new identity and be sure to write down a few of your own as well:

- ★ family, friends and loved ones
- ★ my physical, emotional and mental health
- ★ my soberish journey
- ★ being a good leader and team player in my career
- ★ eating healthy, nutritious food the fuels my body
- ★ getting enough restful sleep and practising good sleep hygiene
- ★ being of service to the soberish community

- ★ ....
- ★ ....
- ★ ....
- ★ ....
- ★ ....

Values: Separate to your priorities, your values are the fundamental beliefs that guide you through the world. Our values can be aligned with our ethics, what kind of person we want to be, how we treat ourselves and others and how we want to show up in the world. Our personal values help us discern between right and wrong and navigate our decision-making. Some common values you may be familiar with or hold are:

- ★ loyalty
- ★ spirituality
- ★ humility
- ★ compassion
- ★ honesty
- ★ kindness
- ★ integrity
- ★ selflessness
- ★ discipline
- ★ dependability
- ★ growth
- ★ generosity
- ★ courage
- ★ gratitude
- ★ wellbeing
- ★ sustainability

For this part of the exercise, it can be particularly helpful to first write out five to ten values you want to hold moving forward, and to then look backward and write down the values you have currently been living by.

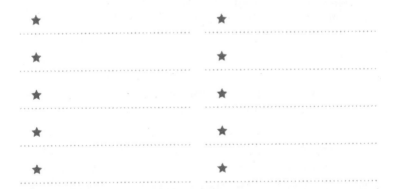

Do you already live by any values that you are proud of? Write down those parts of your current identity you currently value and would like to continue to do so. Where are there any areas for improvement?

Again, remember we won't just be changing our entire value system overnight: this takes time. What we can do is start with a specific new core value that we would like to exude and begin to work on that, like being more honest in our day-to-day life, or exuding more kindness by doing one nice thing a day for someone with no intention of reciprocation.

Pro tip: If you have a hard time pinning down your values, it can be helpful to ask a friend how they perceive you and your values. Have your friend give you some examples of how you have shown those values in the past. Sometimes an outside perspective can help us see the blind spots we may be missing.

Goals: We don't have to dive too deep into goal-setting right now since we've already covered this in chapter 4, but it may be helpful to go back and re-read the section "Design the Life You Want" on pages 73–5 to refresh your memory. Having SMART goals can really set you up for success in your soberish journey and can help you gain awareness into the types of new goals you want to be setting. For example, we want to set goals that reflect our new identity, values and priorities. Perhaps this means focusing on a promotion at work, running a marathon, achieving a soberish milestone of a certain number of alcohol-free days, or setting new boundaries. Whatever the new goal is, the most important question you should ask yourself when setting it is: "Will this goal help me to obtain the new identity I am building for myself? Will it bring me closer to the highest version of myself?" If the answer is yes, you're on the right track. If the answer is no, it's best to trim the fat and let go of nonessential goals that are not currently serving your higher purpose.

One of the most beautiful things about being human is our capacity to adapt to change and build resilience. Just knowing that you are capable of making these big life changes, even if you don't feel confident yet, can be the foundation on which you build your new identity. Maybe you recognize that a lot of your current identity and social connections revolve around alcohol – and that's OK because you are capable of changing your narrative. Simply by having awareness that you want to make change is a huge first step in recreating your identity. As soberish grapevine member Raquel explains:

> *Removing alcohol from my life has allowed me space to learn who I am, and enjoy things I like. I've gained confidence to be silly and loud, and who I truly am. I can now show myself grace and forgiveness. I used to shame myself when I thought about the past or my drinking. I accept it now, I did what I needed to survive. I'm choosing better for myself now since I know better. Show yourself grace. You fuck up, and that's OK. You have to learn to get back up, and keep going. Whatever re-evaluating your relationship with alcohol looks like for you, just acknowledging you want to change it, that's a huge deal! Celebrate everything.*

Once you have acknowledged that you want to change, you can actively look for people who model the sort of qualities that you want to embody – but remember that this isn't about imitating anybody else. This is about shedding old, outdated identities and becoming the amazing individual you were always meant to be before booze started to get in the way.

FIND YOUR OWN ROLE MODEL

Consider someone in your life or someone you admire that radiates the confidence, values and lifestyle you desire. What is it exactly about this person or persons that you admire? What is it about them that you'd like to emulate: their lifestyle, their soberish journey, their self-discipline, their work ethic?

Take time to make a list of thoughtful questions and really consider what it is about this person you desire to emulate. If it's someone you know, consider giving them a call or setting a coffee date to pick their brain.

We all started somewhere, so even if it feels intimidating to reach out to this person, I'm sure they will be more than flattered and happy to speak with you about their personal journey.

IDENTITY BUILDING: BRICK BY BRICK

Using the exercises from the last section, I want you to pin down who you want to be moving forward. Imagine yourself as a blank canvas and compile the priorities, values, goals and characteristics of the person you admire on to this page. This list will be the foundation for your new identity. Below, write down the characteristics of your new, reclaimed identity:

FOSTERING OUR OWN HAPPINESS SANS BOOZE

It is my belief that in order for us to accept ourselves and truly maintain our new lifestyle and identity we must be able to foster and then sustain our own happiness without alcohol. Creating a new identity is a marathon, not a sprint, so if you aren't careful you can fall into the trap of putting in the hard work at the beginning and then falling off. For many of us, this is why habit change hasn't worked well in the past. You make a commitment to do (or not do) something, put in 110 per cent for a month and burn yourself out. The trick is to pace yourself.

I personally do this by practicing the principles described in psychologist Carol Ryff's Model of Psychological Well-Being.[2] To understand Ryff's theory, you first must understand what psychological wellbeing (PWB) is and why it is important. At its most basic level, psychological wellbeing is a core feature of our emotional health and can refer to our positive mental states such as pleasure, fulfilment and proper emotional regulation. Having higher PWB can help us to lead healthier, more satisfying lives. This is especially important when it comes to avoiding backslides, because if we are maintaining high levels of PWB there will be no reason to go back to old unhealthy behaviours. Ryff's Model of Psychological Well-Being breaks down psychological wellbeing into six components that, if maintained, will lead you to taking back your power and learning to foster your own happiness and create an internal locus of control. Here are descriptions of the components so that you can start applying them to your own life too.

1. SELF-ACCEPTANCE

- ★ Someone who has high levels of self-acceptance will possess a positive attitude toward their self, accept both the good and bad qualities they possess and not dwell on the past.
- ★ Someone with low levels of self-acceptance will feel dissatisfied with themselves, be unable to accept all aspects of their personality and often wish to be someone else.

How you can strengthen your self-acceptance:
Self-acceptance can be a truly difficult concept for many of us to grasp. I have struggled with it my entire life and although today I can proudly say I feel I live on the higher end of the spectrum, I still have days and even weeks when I'm filled with self-doubt. I personally found the first step toward self-acceptance was neutrality. Not self-love, not toxic positivity, nor attempting to achieve a clean slate, but looking myself in the mirror and saying, "All right, Kayla, this is what we're working with and that's OK, we build up from here." Simply accepting the fact you aren't where you want to be *yet* but acknowledging you will find a way

to get there can be a big step toward adopting a more positive attitude toward yourself and your past. It sounds a bit clichéd but telling yourself that the only person and thing you control in this world is yourself can be a daily reminder to accept the things you can't change. You can't change the past, nor who you were yesterday, but you can choose a new attitude and outlook on life moving forward. Practising the goal-setting we have talked about can be a big confidence-booster when it comes to learning higher levels of self-acceptance. Setting and achieving attainable goals will help you build self-esteem, which will give you a more positive attitude toward yourself.

2. ENVIRONMENTAL MASTERY

★ Someone with high environmental mastery will have a good sense of managing the environment that they are in, both taking on challenges as these come along and being open to new opportunities. They are able to create an environment that fits their needs and values.

★ Someone with low environmental mastery feels a lack of control over the world around them and has difficulty managing their day-to-day affairs. They may be unaware of surrounding opportunities and feel helpless to their environment.

How to improve your environmental mastery

Life is complex. The truth of the matter is that we often have zero control over other people and their actions but we do have control over our own behaviours. We can start to master the environment we are in by meeting the demands of each situation that is presented to us, rather than becoming overwhelmed by them. For example, I've already mentioned how I am currently writing this book, having experienced some major upheaval. Instead of allowing the situation to overwhelm me, I have used the tools given to you in this book to cope with my own stress and changes of environments. I took on all of these amazing opportunities, and adapted and adjusted to them, even when it wasn't convenient for me at all. Learning to use your new, healthy coping skills to adapt to situations and new environments is how you will improve your environmental mastery. I'm not implying it will be comfortable, but remember that if it doesn't challenge you it doesn't change you.

3. PERSONAL GROWTH

- ★ Someone with high personal growth sees themselves as always evolving. They are open-minded and always looking for ways to improve themselves and gain more knowledge of self.
- ★ Someone with low personal growth feels stagnant, and may have a difficult time changing their self-identity or lifestyle. They are uninterested in changing their current behaviours and attitudes.

How to unleash your full potential through personal growth

You're here reading this book because you want to grow as a person and change old patterns of behaviour to reach your highest potential. I want to reiterate that's a major step in the stages of change and you should be proud of yourself for getting here. We have already covered many of the best tips for personal growth in past chapters, with examples including activities such as visualization, meditation and goal-setting. All of these tools can help you to look toward the future you desire and design a POA strategy to reach your goals. Continuing to be resilient on your journey is also an important part of personal growth. This isn't a linear journey; slips and backslides may occur for many people. It's critical you remind yourself that experiencing old patterns of behaviour is by no means the same as failing – it's a learning opportunity for you to dig deeper and pull out those prickly pears of painful thoughts and feelings you may have missed. No matter what your final destination is, when it comes to your relationship with alcohol, know that this process is non-binary, so if your journey looks like a giant squiggly line in the beginning then you're doing just fine – you're learning to crawl before you walk. As soberish grapevine member Ashley explains:

> When I was drinking, I couldn't trust myself at all. I didn't follow through on promises to myself, and I only followed through on promises to others out of a sense of responsibility. I was really used to letting myself down. Since taking an extended break from booze, I can count on myself to do things that are good for me – anything from having a skincare routine to resisting toxic friendships and relationships. I think I've absolutely experienced personal growth since changing my relationship with alcohol. I'm able to regulate my emotions better, and just make better choices about what matters to me. For me at least, drinking made it really hard to evaluate what was happening around me, and now I can make better choices.

4. POSITIVE RELATIONS WITH OTHERS

★ Someone with high positive relations will have satisfying and deep connections with others. They tend to have high levels of empathy for others and are good listeners.

★ Someone with low positive relations has a hard time giving their trust to others. They tend not to have a large group of friends, and prefer to isolate rather than compromise for their relationships to work.

How to foster positive relations with others

Relationships are hard, especially when you're making a big lifestyle change like drinking less or quitting altogether. Sometimes we realize a lot of our social life has been built around alcohol, or that it feels difficult for us to connect with others without the social lubricant of a few drinks. The good news is there are so many tools available to you to develop positive relationships (new and old) while you navigate improving your wellbeing. Some of these may seem obvious but they are foundational, the first of which is that you need to focus on developing your communication skills. This will help you with all aspects of your life, but especially your relationships. So many fights, resentments and negative situations can be chalked up to simple miscommunication or lack of any communication at all. Recognizing and helping others understand where you are coming from without becoming defensive or upset is a great way to foster healthier connections. This works the other way around as well: be a good listener. And I don't mean just listen and wait for someone to stop talking so you can get a word in, I mean truly aiming to understand what that person is trying to say. A great technique I was taught in couple's therapy actually helped me a lot in this arena, which I am going to share with you now.

●●

LISTEN AND REPEAT

Sometimes we can find ourselves caught up in conversations that quickly escalate into arguments, with each person loudly repeating themselves over and over. Here is a simple practice that you can use to avoid this happening.

★ Sit down with the person you need to talk to in a level-headed, neutral environment.

★ Let them know there is something you need to communicate to them and ask them to listen without judgement.

★ Before you tell them what you want to say, ask them to repeat back to you afterwards what it is that you said. For example, you might say: "Steve, the way you acted last night in front of our friends really hurt my feelings. It felt very much like I wasn't even there. I feel like this is a pattern when we go out. I would really like to be more included when it comes to conversations and activities with your friends. I think it will help strengthen our relationship." Then Steve answers, "So my understanding of what you just said was ..."

★ This exercise will help you to avoid miscommunication because you can have the person reiterate right back to you what you said in that moment and in this way understand their perspective. Perhaps you're on the same page – great! But maybe what Steve heard was that he was a bad boyfriend, even though that isn't what you said. So make sure to reiterate your true message back to the person after they have finished mirroring you: "Steve, I see how you could see it that way, but what I'm really saying is . . ."

★ Once you have spoken your piece, the other person has mirrored this back to you, and you have responded, give them the opportunity to tell you their point of view in the same way, and then repeat their words back to them.

★ Keep the tone neutral and respectful. If the exchange doesn't appear to be working, calmly draw the conversation to a close.

5. PURPOSE IN LIFE

★ Someone with high self-purpose has set goals and feels a strong sense of direction for where they want to go in life. They also hold beliefs and values that give them a higher sense of purpose and meaning.

★ Someone with low self-purpose lacks direction and may feel they have no or little purpose in life. They do not have goals in place to set them up for future success.

How to find purpose in life

This can seem like a tall order, and in a lot of ways it is. But our purpose in life can A) be many things and B) does not have to be about changing the world.

Focusing on the essential is key to fostering happiness through purpose. What do you value and prioritize? (Remember that we've already gone over this!) How can you contribute in a meaningful yet attainable way? It can also be fun to vision-board this idea, get creative and think outside the box. I found my purpose in life through service to others. It was never something I had focused on while I was drinking, but it was a new concept that was introduced to me when I first stopped. The original idea was to simply help out my community in any way I was asked, which I was happy to do, but when I left traditional programming I felt I lacked purpose because I no longer had a community to serve, so I built a new one: 1,000 Hours Dry, aka The Dry Club, and then the Reframe app. As I continue to evolve I find new ways to serve others directly, like this book, the soberish community and my new career at Drink Monday, working to create a cultural shift around non-alcoholic spirits and healthier lifestyles.

6. AUTONOMY

★ Someone with high autonomy can regulate their emotions well and is able to resist social pressure. They feel confident in their independence and live by their own set of standards.

★ Someone with low autonomy is constantly worried about what others think of them and relies on the judgements and expectations of others to live their lives. They are quick to conform to societal norms.

How you can strengthen your autonomy

Autonomy means aligning yourself with people, places and things that allow you to feel confident in your decision-making. When you are on the soberish journey, this requires change. You may need to remove yourself from certain environments, relationships and even work situations. This can be difficult but remember that you are putting yourself first, and setting yourself up for success. The Law of Attraction tells us we attract what we put out, so the more you are surrounded by people and environments that respect your boundaries and champion your independence, the more easily you will be able to build higher levels of autonomy. There is no ceiling to this growth, so continue to seek out opportunities and challenges that allow you to strengthen your autonomy in your personal life, at work and in social settings. Like a muscle that you can hypertrophy, autonomy gets stronger with practice; and the more skills you aim to learn, the more confidence you will ultimately gain in new areas of your life.

Our aim here is to be high in all areas to achieve maximum happiness and wellbeing. This is by no means an overnight process but by focusing on one factor at a time, you can begin to develop tools and skills to become stronger in each category. You may also find that learning the ways to build one factor will help leverage you to foster the others in a quicker fashion. For example, the better you become at practising self-acceptance, the easier it will be for you to find purpose and direction in life.

BUILDING BLOCKS FOR A NEW LIFE

By working one step at a time through this chapter, and all the others before it, you will now have the key ingredients to start building a new you who is no longer in thrall to alcohol. You hopefully have a much clearer sense of the priorities, values and goals that you want to place at the centre of your life, and you can start to see ways to make the issues that are truly important to you part of your everyday reality.

You will also be more aware of the importance of fostering your own happiness through the six components that lead to psychological wellbeing. While you will know that your soberish journey might not be easy, that there will likely be setbacks and backslides along the way, and not everyone will be supportive, it's hopefully becoming a little clearer each day that you are on the brink of an incredible adventure – a wonderful life is out there, waiting for you to enjoy it.

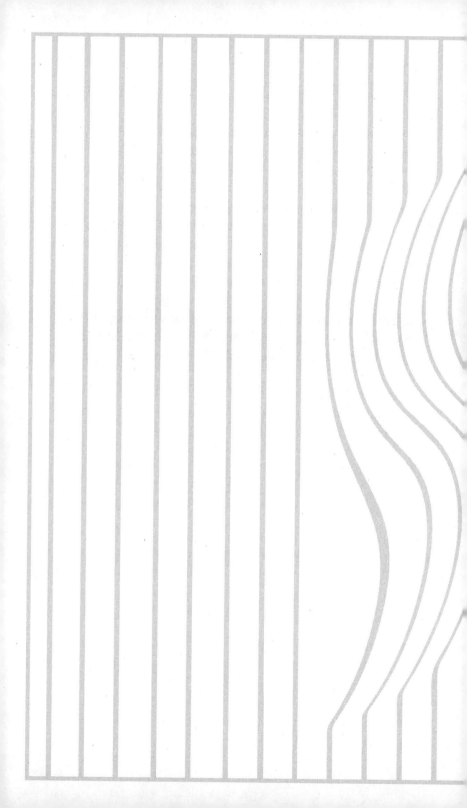

CHAPTER 17

Ready, Set, Show Time

Here we are. It's almost show time. *Are you ready?*
Because you now have everything you need to start
building the foundation for your new soberish lifestyle.
Everything we've gone over together has purposefully
focused on building and improving your internal locus
of control – from newfound knowledge, to a plethora
of holistic tools for coping with stressors and cravings,
and, most importantly, for creating a new mindset.
Even if you're scared of change, that's OK: it's good
to be afraid sometimes; it means you're getting out
of your comfort zone. Nothing new can grow while
you are stuck in there.

Now that you've stepped outside of that bubble and
into a land of endless opportunities, it's time to prepare
you with a few last tips before the red curtain rises.
Changing your relationship with alcohol, no matter
what that looks like, will present its own unique
challenges, but the beauty of the transformation you're
choosing to undergo is that you will only get stronger
and more resilient over time in order to face them
head on. Life will continue to happen as it always has.
Tragedies will occur, moments of social anxiety will
come and go, heartbreak will test your willpower,
but through it all you will stay strong because you
now have the tools to take on the world.

I myself have experienced more adversity and
uncomfortable situations in the last seven years while
on my journey than I had in my entire life until then.
From being in a domestically violent relationship and
leaving it, surviving a horrendous motorcycle accident,
losing friends to overdoses, to facing my social anxiety
head on, going on first dates dead-ass sober and
trimming the fat off friendships that no longer served
me, I endured and overcame it all. And so can you.

Had I been drinking during any of those times, I can
only imagine how much worse each of those situations

would have been. Would I have had the clear mind and courage to leave someone who was hurting me? Could I have been the friend others needed to lean on during their own grief and heartbreak? Could I have had the grace and resilience to pick myself up off the floor, literally, and start over, rather than beg someone to stay with me where I wasn't wanted? Would I have seen the red flags that were normally blurred by rosé-coloured glasses? The simple answer is *no*.

So while drinking may have been the easy way to escape the pain or discomfort of many different situations, I'm not one to do things the easy way. I have learned that the only way out of challenges is through them. That in order to get rid of all of your prickly pears of negativity, hurt and suffering, you must pick them out, one by one, no matter the discomfort, the anxiety or the fear it brings you. Because the only thing more terrifying than facing our fears, is continuing to live life the way that we have been, never changing.

I know I've stated this a million times, but I'm going to say it again: this journey isn't linear. Backslides and old behaviours may rear their ugly heads, but that doesn't mean you aren't making progress. Remember the tortoise and the hare? Yeah – not everything in life is about going fast. It's about going at your own pace. Remember that you're building a completely new foundation. If you were building a house, would you want the construction workers to pour the cement foundation in as quickly as possible just to get it done, or would you rather have them take their time, smoothing the edges, making sure to fix any cracks that may occur and adding an extra layer for care? Probably the latter.

So think of your foundation in the same way. It's OK to have cracks: take the time to smooth them over and figure out why they happened so you don't make the same mistake twice. Go at your own pace; the only person you need to be worried about being "better than" is yesterday's version of you. Comparing your progress to that of others will only throw you off course. We all have different timelines and paths that aren't meant to be parallel. So if this means you need to unfollow certain people on social media or distance yourself from people who don't support that, *do you*.

Once you have solidified your foundation, the rest of this journey is all about building that dream life, the one you have always deserved, and then maintaining it. You do this brick by brick. Each day you wake up and put in the effort toward becoming your highest self is a day you put a new brick into the wall. When backslides happen, you simply reflect and don't put a brick in the wall that day. Again, progress here isn't linear; there may be days or weeks where you feel stagnant or turn to old behaviours out of habit or fear.

Just remember that everything you have built is already there for you, and slipping up doesn't mean taking a sledgehammer to your wall or foundation – it just means you don't get to put a brick in that day. If you were running a marathon and tripped, would you go back to the start line? Absolutely not. Or what if (God forbid) you get some mascara on your top lid after you've already done your eye makeup? Are you going to take off the whole eye and start over? *No, you aren't a psychopath!* You take a damn Q-tip and wipe off the mascara.

We've been programmed to believe that this whole process of changing our relationship with alcohol is binary, but it isn't. So no matter what you decide to do after reading this book, know that all of the knowledge you've gained by reading it is somewhere in your subconscious brain. You have planted a seed deep in your mind and it will not fall out of your head just because you pick up a drink.

ENTER THE ANTAGONIST: DEALING WITH CHALLENGES, DRY

I had the absolute privilege of speaking with so many unique individuals on all points of the soberish spectrum throughout the process of writing this book – from those who now drink mindfully after a stint with problematic drinking, to the sober-curious, to those in recovery and everyone in between. It feels important for me not just to give my own advice and outlook but to share as many experiences as possible, as I am only one person with a single perspective. That's why I've asked people I trust to help me with this last bit, and that's the show time itself – those real-life scenarios that most of us will face at some point in our soberish journey. It amazes me that no matter the background or circumstance, so many of you have the same questions and want advice on the same topics. I hope the following topics, questions and answers will give you deeper insight and encouragement to know that you've got this in the bag.

How did you manage not drinking and/or starting your soberish journey during college?

Personally, I didn't stop drinking when I was in college, although I wish I had as it would have saved me a lot of embarrassment and money. But I did know I had a problem, even before college. It unfortunately took a court-ordered trip to rehab to really open my eyes to the gravity of the situation I had put myself in. I hope that you haven't had to dig yourself that deep in order to be here, but even if you have, there is always a way out. When I was in school there were little to no resources given to students outside of sending us to the counselling office or a local town AA meeting. And what 20-year-old wants to admit they're an alcoholic? Probably none. But the beautiful thing today is that there are more resources available than ever. Colleges and universities have their own Collegiate Recovery Programs (CRC), and there are special support groups just for young people, like the online group Steady Sundays or Young People in Recovery (YPIR). Soberish grapevine member Stephanie S., a friend and YouTuber, explained to me how her college supported her in quitting:

> College was the perfect place for me to hide my drinking problem. Suddenly, all the thoughts I'd been having for years about whether or not my drinking was healthy were suddenly silenced by the normalized, binge-drinking culture I saw all around me. But after years of embarrassment, guilt, and harm to my mind and body, I knew I needed to make a change.
>
> I started seeing a counsellor at my school to talk about how to cut back on my drinking. Through talking with him, I started to realize the extent of my drinking issues. The blackouts, the hangovers, the sneaking drinks, the drinking alone. These were not "normal behaviours". This counsellor was the first person ever in my life to suggest the idea of sobriety.
>
> After working with him for a month or two, I finally realized that alcohol could not be a part of my life. My options were to deal with it while still in college, or deal with it in 5, 10, or 15 years' time. Once I finally concluded that there would never be a "perfect time" to give up alcohol and get sober, I made the commitment to try it out. I aimed to protect my sobriety at all costs.
>
> For me, this meant going into a "hibernation" mode and avoiding all activities and events that may have been triggering my drinking. This meant leaving events ASAP if I got any indication that I may want to drink. Of course, I struggled with this at times, and there were

quite a few moments where I spent way too long at an event that was testing my sobriety, but for the most part, putting my sobriety above anything else in my life for the first few months was crucial.

Being completely honest with the people in my life that I was close to and spent a lot of time with about why I quit drinking was important and helpful as well. For me, it was a bit different because I was so vocal about my sobriety on social media that I didn't really need to explain to very many people why I wasn't drinking, but that didn't happen until later on. When I first got sober, it was crucial for me to tell my roommates so that they knew my goals and how to best support me.

According to research, Gen Z is drinking 20 per cent less than millennials, who are also drinking less than both Gen X and Boomers.[1] There's a cultural shift at large happening where drinking less is becoming more and more normalized and it's not going anywhere.

How do you deal with peer pressure from others to drink or drink more than you want?

Similar to having a complete soberish toolkit, it's important we each have our own tiny toolkit for dealing with certain situations such as peer pressure. While you may not be able to start meditating in the middle of a party or bar when you're feeling like drinking, you can try using other tactics to overcome the challenge of peer pressure. One of my favourite tips is from my friend Maggie B., who suggests "always having a quick one-off response about why you're not drinking in your back pocket, and sticking to it. For me, 'My life is better without alcohol', or, 'I stopped liking who I became when I drank' are pretty solid, simple answers that usually shut up even the most pressuring of people."

Other times avoiding the scenario altogether if you aren't quite ready is totally OK too! If you don't feel 100 per cent confident, don't put yourself at risk. There's a difference between doing things that scare us and putting ourselves in harm's way. When I first stopped drinking, I didn't go out much and planned a lot of non-alcohol-centric gatherings with my friends who also didn't drink. The luxury of this idea is that you don't have to have other non-drinking or soberish friends to participate in activities that don't involve drinking, just put together a boozeless brunch or a yoga class and invite whoever you'd like. Your friends who don't respect your new boundaries will weed out quickly. Like my friend Melissa E. says: "It helps to keep in mind that it's a 'them' problem and not a 'you' problem. I realized early on that typically the people who tried to pressure you to drink, or were uncomfortable with the fact that you weren't, was because they were insecure with their own drinking habits."

How do you navigate "dry dating"?

I am personally a big fan of dry dating. When you drink, you tend to lower your inhibitions and miss red flags you may have picked up on while you were sober. I also realized I can connect with my date on a much deeper level when I'm dry, I'm able to tell if the attraction is real and listen to what my intuition is telling me about the person. In general, I also tend to make better decisions that align with my values, while when I was drinking I may have lowered my standards or even slept with someone I normally wouldn't because of the "beer goggle" effect.

The trick is to choose environments for the first few dates that don't centre around alcohol. This could be grabbing coffee or juice, going for a walk, mini-golf, seeing a movie or doing something active.

"Be upfront!" explains my girlfriend Melissa, who stopped drinking at age 22. "I always tell people very early on that I'm sober. If you're new to sobriety or don't feel comfortable sharing that you struggle with AUD, you can just say you don't feel like drinking or you can't drink on medicine, etc. Usually when I tell people that I'm sober they're really impressed and want to know more. It depends on the situation but usually if they have questions I'll go into more detail!" My friend Kate G. had similar advice: "For those navigating 'app dating', I always let people know that I didn't drink before we met up for the date. This ensures that I am not wasting my time on someone who might judge me for not drinking. I always tried to plan a date that did not revolve around alcohol. For example: going for a walk, having dinner, coffee, etc."

How do you navigate new friends and new activities that don't revolve around drinking?

It was rough at first – eventually I had to get honest with myself and accept others' opinions about my choice; their attitudes to my not drinking have nothing to do with me and more with them and their relationship with alcohol. As far as finding a new community, the best answer I could give and what many of my friends suggested was social media, and local sober-curious groups. Rachel suggests finding friends "by looking up local sober groups on Instagram". She adds: "I found one in my city. The girls were so comforting and helped validate my feelings so I didn't feel alone. Outside of the sober community, I think it helps to focus on activities that light you up, whether that's yoga, journaling, hiking, pottery, etc. and finding groups that host events in your area or online." (Rachel and I actually met through Instagram and have become great friends IRL from our Orange County women's group, OCSBC!)

"One way to find new activities that don't revolve around drinking is to think about everything you enjoyed before your first drink," explains Kate G. "For example, I was a competitive runner in high school, and sobriety gave me the energy to work out. I currently attend weekly workout classes with friends. I also love reading, colouring books and cooking."

I myself took exercise back up, as well as creative outlets like vision-boarding and reading. It took a little while to fully enjoy the activities in the same way because of anhedonia (see page 12), but over time my brain readjusted and I was able to find pleasure in hobbies outside drinking. Steph S. had a similar experience:

> I really dove into things that I used to enjoy doing, but "grew out of" once peer pressure convinced me that drinking was the "cool" thing to do now. This included reading, scrapbooking and hiking. Sobriety also gave me the courage to start a YouTube channel to channel my creativity. This is something that I had been wanting to do for a decade but never had the confidence or time to do because of how insecure drinking made me. Sobriety allows you to take a clear look at your life and truly go after what you want!

TIME TO LIVE THE LIFE YOU HAVE ALWAYS DESERVED

It's one thing to read the pages of a book and theorize about imaginary scenarios, and quite another to encounter situations in RL that could challenge your commitment to staying the course of your soberish journey – but you've got this. Know that there are countless people around the world who have already faced, or who will go on to face, the same sort of obstacles and setbacks that may come up for you on your soberish journey. Reach out to those people. A supportive community is a tool that is definitely worth having to hand, whether or not you decide to include other tools like breathwork or cold treatments in your POA.

And be prepared for all eventualities by creating your own unique set of mini tools, especially designed for dealing with situations that are likely to come up for you – like those Friday office drinks, peer pressure in the college bar, or that well-meaning relative who always presses a glass in your hand as they're used to you being their drinking buddy. Say as much as you need to say, but don't ever think you need to apologize to anybody else for choosing to set aside your old habits, practise self-care and live the life you deserve.

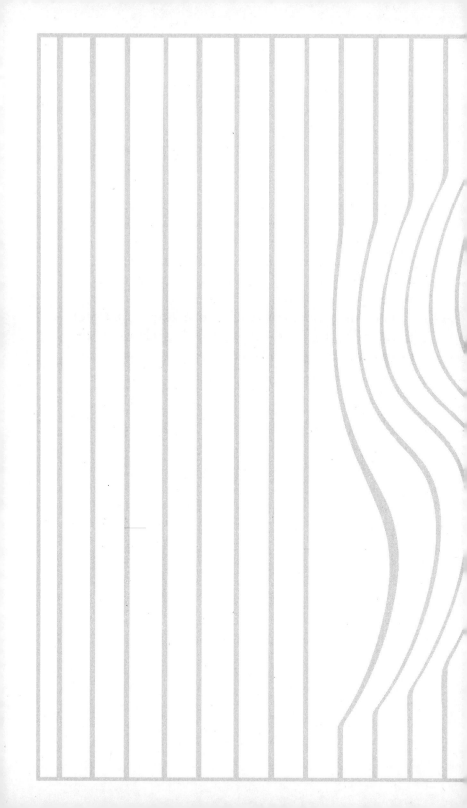

Conclusion:
Welcome to
a Soberish
Way of Life

CONCLUSION: WELCOME TO A SOBERISH WAY OF LIFE

Congratulations – I am so proud of you for deciding to read this book and making it this far on your soberish journey! You have shown that you have the willingness and the courage to change, and there's a new life waiting for you because of the choices that you are making each day. Soberish is about intention and freedom, not restriction; it's about the pleasures of regaining control of our lives and enjoying so much more than alcohol could ever offer us in the first place.

The brain's neuroplasticity means that while our old drinking patterns may have become unhelpful habits, we are capable of rewiring our thinking. This doesn't involve willpower, shame or blame; it's about taking back your narrative, looking after your key physical and mental needs – and having powerful tools at your disposal that will help you to realign yourself with your priorities, values and goals. You don't need to hit rock bottom to choose sobriety, or need to define yourself with labels like "alcoholic" or "AUD"; all you have to do is to be willing to question your relationship with alcohol. It's about knowing that there is more out there waiting for you, and it's about waking up without a hangover and loving life.

The soberish journey invites you to create a fulfilling vision for your future and reclaim your power from booze so that you can make that vision of yours a reality. This won't be a linear process; there will be backslides, setbacks and surprises – there may even be times when you feel like you have completely lost your way – but any progress you make will never be wasted. Each day offers a fresh opportunity to live your best life, and there is a whole community of likeminded soberish individuals out there waiting for you to join them and ready to support you every step of the way.

Resources

You will find details of supportive online communities on pages 215–16. I've refrained from sharing the details of other organizations who can help with alcohol issues here, as I'm reluctant to recommend anything that I haven't tried myself. However, there are tons of groups out there, so I would encourage you to do some research into those local to you – and please think about joining the soberish community, the details of which you will find below.

Body Intuition:
Nikita Mehta, grey area drinking coach, yoga instructor RYT 200
Instagram: @nikitakmehta

Cold Exposure:
Marcus Bradley, level-two Wim Hof method instructor
Instagram: @thebreathinvegan
Website: www.wimhofmethod.com/instructors/marcus-bradley

Conscious Manifestation:
Emma Mumford, manifestation expert and author of *Positively Wealthy*
Instagram: @iamemmamumford
Website: www.emmamumford.co.uk

Meditation and Intuitive Movement:
Lindsay Dalton, trauma-informed breathwork facilitator and yoga and meditation instructor RYT 200
Instagram: @_lindsaydalton

Nutrition and Gut Health:
Dr Brooke Scheller, doctor of nutrition and creator
of "Functional Sobriety"
Instagram @drbrookescheller
Website: www.brookescheller.com

Dr Jeff Simone, doctor of pharmacy, Certified Advanced
Dietary Supplement Adviser and creator of Reaction
Recovery
Instagram: @reactionrecovery
Website: www.reactionrecovery.com

Soberish Community:
Kayla Lyons, Instagram @kaylerlyons
Soberish, Instagram @joinsoberish

Sound Therapy:
Farzana Ali, sound therapist and author
Instagram @thesoundtherapist
Summer Muse, sound healer
Instagram @soundwithsummer or @thesummermuse

Tackling Domestic Abuse:
National Domestic Violence Hotline (US)
Tel: 800.799.SAFE (7233)
Website: www.thehotline.org
1800 Respect (AU)
The National Sexual Assault, Family & Domestic
Violence Counselling Service
Tel: 1800 737 732
Website: www.1800respect.org.au
Refuge's National Domestic Abuse Helpline (UK):
Tel: 0808 2000 247
Women's Aid (UK)
Website: helpline@womensaid.org.uk

Endnotes

Introduction

1   See Ana María Rosso (2012). "Beer and Wine in Antiquity: Beneficial Remedy or Punishment Imposed by the Gods?", *Acta med-hist Adriat*, 10(2), pp.237–262. Available at: hrcak.srce.hr/file/141909

2   See Iain Gately (2009). *Drink: A Cultural History of Alcohol*. New York: Gotham Books.

3   Ibid.

4   See Ellen Castlow (n.d.). "Mother's Ruin", Historic UK website. Available at: www.historic-uk.com/CultureUK/Mothers-Ruin/ (Accessed: 26 Jan 2023.)

5   For more information, see, for example: en.wikipedia.org/wiki/Gin_Act_1751

6   See British Library (n.d.). "Temperance card", British Library website.

7   See Jack S. Blocker, Jr. (2006 February). "Did Prohibition Really Work? Alcohol Prohibition as a Public Health Innovation", *Am J Public Health*, 96(2), pp. 233–43. DOI: 10.2105/AJPH.2005.065409

8   Code of Federal Regulations (24 Jan 2023). Title 27, eCFR website. Available at: www.ecfr.gov/current/title-27/chapter-I/subchapter-A/part-16 (Accessed: 26 Jan 2023.)

9   Centres for Disease Control and Prevention (n.d.), "Alcohol Use and Your Health", CDC website. Available at: www.cdc.gov/alcohol/fact-sheets/alcohol-use.htm (Accessed: 26 Jan 2023.)

10 Anna Blackwell (15 Nov, 2017), "What eye-tracking told us about alcohol warning labels in the UK", Alcohol Labelling website. Available at: labelling.blogs.bristol.ac.uk/2017/11/15/what-eye-tracking-told-us-about-alcohol-warning-labels-in-the-uk/

11 See Blocker, "Did Prohibition Really Work? Alcohol Prohibition as a Public Health Innovation".

12 Ibid.

13 Ibid.

14 See Barbara Ellen (24 Jul 2022). "Gen Z for zero tolerance: why British youth are turning off booze", *Guardian*. Available at: www.theguardian.com/society/2022/jul/24/

gen-z-for-zero-tolerance-why-british-youth-are-turning-off-booze (Accessed 7 Mar 2023.)

15 See Katie Hunt (12 Oct 2020). "Young Americans more likely to say no to alcohol, study finds", CNN website. Available at: edition.cnn.com/2020/10/12/health/young-adults-drinking-less-alcohol-us-wellness/index.html (Accessed 7 Mar 2023.)

16 Sarah Gardner and Dave Albee (2015). "Study focuses on strategies for achieving goals, resolutions". Press Releases. 266. Available at: scholar.dominican.edu/news-releases/266 (Accessed: 8 Feb 2023.)

1. Understanding the Brain–Booze Connection

1 Author interview with Gillian Tietz on Zoom (16 Dec, 2022).

2 See also Health Promotion and Disease Prevention Knowledge Gateway (31 May 2022). "National low-risk drinking recommendations (or drinking guidelines) and standard units", European Commission website. Available at: knowledge4policy.ec.europa.eu/health-promotion-knowledge-gateway/national-low-risk-drinking-recommendations-drinking-guidelines_en (Accessed: 7 Mar 2023.)

3 See Kim Bloomfield, Tim Stockwell, Gerhard Gmel and Nina Rehn (n.d.). "International Comparisons of Alcohol Consumption", National Institute on Alcohol Abuse website. Available at: pubs.niaaa.nih.gov/publications/arh27-1/95-109.htm (Accessed: 30 Jan 2023.)

4 The Athlete (n.d.). "Drug Abuse: Absorption, Distribution, & Metabolism", The Athlete website. Available at: www.theathlete.org/drug-abuse/absorption.htm (Accessed: 31 Jan 2023.)

5 Claire Sissons (27 May 2020). "What is the average percentage of water in the human body?", Medical News Today website. Available at: www.medicalnewstoday.com/articles/what-percentage-of-the-human-body-is-water. (Accessed: 31 Jan 2023.)

6 The Alcohol Pharmacology Education Partnership (n.d.). "Gender Differences in Alcohol Metabolism", Duke University website. Available at: sites.duke.edu/apep/module-1-gender-matters/content/content-gender-differences-in-alcohol-metabolism/

7 See H. A. Carroll, M. K. Lustyk and M. E. Larimer (Dec, 2015). "The relationship between alcohol consumption

and menstrual cycle: a review of the literature", *Arch Womens Ment Health*, 18(6), pp.773–81. DOI: 10.1007/s00737-015-0568-2.

8   See NHS (n.d.). "Risks: alcohol misuse", NHS website. Available at: www.nhs.uk/conditions/alcohol-misuse/risks/ (Accessed: 8 Feb 2023.)

9   Ibid.

10   See Alan Woodruff and Jürgen Götz. (n.d.). "What is the blood-brain barrier?", Queensland Brain Institute website. Available at: qbi.uq.edu.au/brain/brain-anatomy/what-blood-brain-barrier (Accessed: 31 Jan 2023.)

11   Alyssa (n.d.). "Blood-Brain Barrier and Alcohol", Banyan Treatment Centres website. Available at: www.banyantreatmentcenter.com/2020/11/02/blood-brain-barrier-and-alcohol-pompano/ (Accessed: 31 Jan 2023.)

12   Author interview with Gillian Tietz.

13   See "Brain Anatomy – Part 3", My-MS.org website. Available at: my-ms.org/anatomy_brain_part3.htm. (Accessed: 31 Jan 2023.)

14   See Daniel K. Hall-Flavin (n.d.). "Antidepressants and alcohol: what's the concern?", Mayo Clinic website. Available at: www.mayoclinic.org/diseases-conditions/depression/expert-answers/antidepressants-and-alcohol/faq-20058231 (Accessed 31 Jan 2023.)

15   See P. Gorwood (2008). "Neurobiological mechanisms of anhedonia", *Dialogues Clin Neurosci*, 10(3), pp.291–9. DOI: 10.31887/DCNS.2008.10.3/pgorwood.

16   National Institute on Alcohol Abuse and Alcoholism (2020). "Understanding Alcohol Use Disorder", NIAAA website. Available at: www.niaaa.nih.gov/publications/brochures-and-fact-sheets/understanding-alcohol-use-disorder (Accessed: 31 Jan 2023.)

17   Author interview.

18   See Jennifer Berry (12 Jan 2023). "What are neurotransmitters?", MedicalNewsToday website. Available at: www.medicalnewstoday.com/articles/326649 (Accessed: 31 Jan 2023.)

19   See C. Pittenger, M. H. Bloch and K. Williams (Dec 2011). "Glutamate abnormalities in obsessive compulsive disorder: neurobiology, pathophysiology, and treatment", *Pharmacol Ther.*, 132(3), pp.314–32. DOI: 10.1016/j.pharmthera.2011.09.006.

20   Michael H. Bloch, Vladimir Coric and Christopher Pittenger (2009). "New Horizons in OCD Research

and the Potential Importance of Glutamate. Can We Develop Treatments That Work Better and Faster?", International OCD Foundation website. Available at: iocdf.org/expert-opinions/expert-opinion-glutamate/ (Accessed: 31 Jan 2023.)

21   Charles L. Pickens and Donna J. Calu (19 Oct 2011). "Alcohol Reward, Dopamine Depletion, and GDNF", *Journal of Neuroscience*, 31(42), pp. 14833–4; DOI: doi. org/10.1523/JNEUROSCI.4222-11.2011 (Accessed: 31 Jan 2023.)

22   Author interview.

23   See J. M. Boden and D. M. Fergusson (May 2011). "Alcohol and depression", *Addiction*, 106(5), pp.906–14. DOI: 10.1111/j.1360-0443.2010.03351.x.

24   Darryl Inaba (2017). "Diathesis Stress Model of Addiction: Etiology of Substance-Related and Addictive Disorders" (recorded webinar), naadac.org. Available at: www.naadac.org/diathesisstressmodelofaddiction.

25   See V. Vasiliou, et al. (Jan 2006). "CYP2E1 and catalase influence ethanol sensitivity in the central nervous system", *Pharmacogenetics and Genomics*, 16(1), pp. 51–8. DOI: 10.1097/01.fpc.0000182777.95555.56 (Accessed: 1 Feb 2023.)

26   See Samir Zakhari, "Overview: How Is Alcohol Metabolized by the Body?" National Institute on Alcohol Abuse website. Available at: pubs.niaaa.nih.gov/ publications/arh294/245-255.htm. (Accessed: 1 Feb 2023)

27   See H. J. Edenberg and T. Foroud (Aug 2013). "Genetics and alcoholism", *Nat Rev Gastroenterol Hepatol.*, 10(8), pp.487–94. DOI: 10.1038/nrgastro.2013.86.

28   Alcohol Alert (July 2007). "Alcohol Metabolism: An Update", National Institute on Alcohol Abuse website. Available at: pubs.niaaa.nih.gov/publications/aa72/aa72. htm. (Accessed: 1 Feb 2023.)

29   The Alcohol Pharmacology Education Partnership (n.d.), "Gender Differences in Alcohol Metabolism", Duke University website. Available at: sites.duke.edu/apep/ module-1-gender-matters/content/content-gender-differences-in-alcohol-metabolism/

30   E. Mellos, I. Liappas and T. Paparrigopoulos (Sep 2010). "Comorbidity of Personality Disorders with Alcohol Abuse", *In Vivo*, 24(5), pp. 761–769. Available at: iv.iiarjournals.org/content/24/5/761 (Accessed: 1 Feb 2023.)

31   N. M. Bakhshani (Jun 2014). "Impulsivity: a predisposition
      toward risky behaviors", *Int J High Risk Behav Addict*. 1;
      3(2):e20428. DOI: 10.5812/ijhrba.20428. Available at:
      www.ncbi.nlm.nih.gov/pmc/articles/PMC4080475/
      (Accessed: 1 Feb 2023.)
32   HelpGuide (n.d.). "Emotional and Psychological Trauma",
      HelpGuide website. Available at: www.helpguide.org/
      articles/ptsd-trauma/coping-with-emotional-and-
      psychological-trauma.htm (Accessed: 1 Feb 2023.)
33   Karina Margit Erdelyi (31 Aug 2021). "Can Trauma
      Be Passed Down From One Generation to the Next?",
      Psycom website. Available at: www.psycom.net/trauma/
      epigenetics-trauma (Accessed: 1 Feb 2023.)
34   Yale Medicine, "Chronic Stress", Yale Medicine website.
      Available at: www.yalemedicine.org/conditions/stress-
      disorder (Accessed: 1 Feb 2023.)
35   De Falco, Emanuela et al. (Sep 2021). "Impaired
      cognitive flexibility and heightened urgency are
      associated with increased alcohol consumption in
      rodent models of excessive drinking", *Addiction Biology*,
      26(5), p.e13004. Available at: doi.org/10.1111/adb.13004
      (Accessed: 7 Mar 2023.)
36   Anthony A. Mercadante and Prasanna Tadi (July 2022).
      "Neuroanatomy, Gray Matter", National Library of
      Medicine website. Available at: www.ncbi.nlm.nih.gov/
      books/NBK553239/ (Accessed: 1 Feb 2022.)
37   Alcoholism: Clinical & Experimental Research (16 Oct
      2012). "Recovery of brain volumes with abstinence
      may vary for different brain regions," ScienceDaily
      website. Available at: www.sciencedaily.com/
      releases/2012/10/121016163132.htm (Accessed:
      1 Feb 2023.)
38   Author interview.
39   G. D. Goodman et al. (Aug 2019). "Impact of Smoking
      and Alcohol Use on Facial Aging in Women: Results
      of a Large Multinational, Multiracial, Cross-sectional
      Survey", *J Clin Aesthet Dermatol*., 12(8), pp.28–39.
      Available at: www.ncbi.nlm.nih.gov/pmc/articles/
      PMC6715121/ (Accessed: 1 Feb 2023.)

2. Taking Back Your Narrative

1   See A. Vaish, T. Grossmann and A. Woodward
     (May 2008). "Not all emotions are created equal: the
     negativity bias in social-emotional development",

Psychol Bull., 134(3), pp.383–403. DOI: 10.1037/0033-2909.134.3.383. (Accessed: 3 Feb 2023)

2   Charlotte Nickerson (8 Oct 2021). "Labeling Theory", SimplyPsychology website. Available at: www.simplypsychology.org/labeling-theory.html (Accessed: 3 Feb 2023.)

3   Ibid.

4   John F. Kelly and Cassandra M. Westerhoff (2010). "Does it matter how we refer to individuals with substance-related conditions? A randomized study of two commonly used terms", *International Journal of Drug Policy*, 21(3), pp.202–7. Available at: www.sciencedirect.com/science/article/pii/S0955395909001546 (Accessed: 7 Mar 2023.)

3. Finding Answers Through Introspection

1   See NHS (n.d.), "Alcohol Units", NHS website. Available at: www.nhs.uk/live-well/alcohol-advice/calculating-alcohol-units/ (Accessed: 7 Feb 2023.)

2   See NIH (n.d.), "Understanding Binge Drinking", NHS website. Available at: www.niaaa.nih.gov/publications/brochures-and-fact-sheets/binge-drinking

3   Ibid.

4   Vivia McCutcheon (29 Nov 2017). "Alcohol use as a high-risk health behavior", Institute for Public Health website. Available at: publichealth.wustl.edu/alcohol-use-as-a-high-risk-health-behavior/ (Accessed: 8 Feb 2023.)

5   See Molly Triffin (18 Sep 2021), "How Bad Is It Really to Drink Alcohol on an Empty Stomach?", Livestrong.com website. Available at: www.livestrong.com/article/13764706-drinking-on-an-empty-stomach/ (Accessed: 7 Feb 2023.)

6   Susanne Reed (7 Mar 2022). "Eating Disorders and Alcoholism: 41% of People With ED Have an Addiction", Alcoholic Resource Centre website. Available at: alcoholicsanonymous.com/mental-health/alcoholism-and-eating-disorders/ (Accessed: 7 Feb 2023.)

7   See NIH, "The Link Between Stress and Alcohol" (n.d.), *Alcohol Alert*, No.85, NIH website. Available at: pubs.niaaa.nih.gov/publications/AA85/AA85.htm (Accessed: 7 Feb 2023)

8   See Katherine M. Keyes, Mark L. Hatzenbuehler and Deborah S. Hasin (5 Mar 2011). "Stressful life

experiences, alcohol consumption, and alcohol use disorders: the epidemiologic evidence for four main types of stressors", *Psychopharmacology*, 218, pp.1–17. Available at: doi.org/10.1007/s00213-011-2236-1 (Accessed: 7 Feb 2023.)

4. The Keys to Success: Goal-Setting and Preparation

1   See Robert E. Levasseur (2001). "People Skills: Change Management Tools: Lewin's Change Model", *Interfaces* 31(4), pp. 71–3. DOI: 10.1287/inte.31.4.71.9674
2   See an explanation at: cce.bard.edu/files/Setting-Goals.pdf
3   SAMSHA (n.d.). "Setting Goals and Developing Specific, Measurable, Achievable, Relevant, and Time-bound Objectives", SAMSHA website. Available at: www. samhsa.gov/sites/default/files/nc-smart-goals-fact-sheet. pdf (Accessed: 8 Feb 2023.)

5. Eat Well: Nourish Your Body's Second Brain

1   See Faraz Bishehsari, et al. (1 Jan 2017). "Alcohol and Gut-derived Inflammation", Alcohol Research website. Available at: arcr.niaaa.nih.gov/volume/38/2/alcohol-and-gut-derived-inflammation (Accessed: 16 Feb 2023.)
2   See M. I. Butler, et al. (Nov 2019). "The Gut Microbiome and Mental Health: What Should We Tell Our Patients?: Le microbiote Intestinal et la Santé Mentale: que Devrions-Nous dire à nos Patients?", *Can J Psychiatry*, 64(11), pp.747–60. DOI: 10.1177/0706743719874168.
3   Author interview with Dr Brooke Scheller (7 Dec 2022).
4   UCSF (n.d.). "Increasing Fiber Intake", UCSF Health website. Available at: www.ucsfhealth.org/education/increasing-fiber-intake (Accessed: 16 Feb 2023.)
5   Uma Naidoo (8 Jan 2021). "Why Do I Always Crave Sweets When I Give Up Alcohol? MDs Explain", MGBHealth website. Available at: www.mindbodygreen. com/articles/sugar-cravings-after-quitting-alcohol (Accessed: 9 Mar 2023.)
6   C. S. Lieber (2003). "Relationships between nutrition, alcohol use, and liver disease", *Alcohol Res Health*, 27(3), pp.220–31. Available at: www.ncbi.nlm.nih.gov/pmc/articles/PMC6668875/
7   Mayo Clinic Staff (n.d.). "Whole grains: Hearty options for a healthy diet", Mayo Clinic website. Available at:

www.mayoclinic.org/healthy-lifestyle/nutrition-and-healthy-eating/in-depth/whole-grains/art-20047826 (Accessed: 16 Feb 2023.)

8   Private email correspondence with Jeff Simone.

9   NHS (n.d.). "Do I need vitamin supplements?", NHS website. Available at: www.nhs.uk/common-health-questions/food-and-diet/do-i-need-vitamin-supplements/ (Accessed: 16 Feb 2023.)

10   NHS (n.d.). "Water, drinks and your health", NHS website. Available at: www.nhs.uk/live-well/eat-well/food-guidelines-and-food-labels/water-drinks-nutrition/ (Accessed: 17 Feb 2023.)

6. Sleep On It: The Healing Power of Rest

1   Whitehall of Deerfield Healthcare (28 Feb 2022). "5 important ways that sleep helps you heal", Whitehall of Deerfield Healthcare website. Available at: www.whitehallofdeerfield.com/blog/5-important-ways-that-sleep-helps-you-heal/ (Accessed: 17 Feb 2023.)

2   Danielle Pacheco (8 Feb 2022). "Alcohol and Sleep", Sleep Foundation website. Available at: www.sleepfoundation.org/nutrition/alcohol-and-sleep (Accessed: 17 Feb 2023.)

3   Eric Suni (29 Sep 2022). "Sleep Hygiene", Sleep Foundation website. Available at: www.sleepfoundation.org/sleep-hygiene (Accessed: 17 Feb 2023.)

4   Harvard Health Publishing (7 Jul 2022). "Blue light has a dark side", Harvard Health Publishing website. Available at: www.health.harvard.edu/staying-healthy/blue-light-has-a-dark-side (Accessed: 17 Feb 2023.)

5   Eric Suni (8 Feb 2022). "Melatonin and Sleep", Sleep Foundation website. Available at: www.sleepfoundation.org/melatonin (Accessed: 17 Feb 2023.)

6   NHS (n.d.). "Melatonin for sleep problems", NHS website. Available at: www.nhs.uk/medicines/melatonin/ (Accessed: 17 Feb 2023.)

7   Danielle Pacheco (13 Feb 2023). "The Best Temperature for Sleep", Sleep Foundation website. Available at: www.sleepfoundation.org/bedroom-environment/best-temperature-for-sleep (Accessed 17 Feb 2023.)

8   S. Haghayegh et al. (Aug 2019). "Before-bedtime passive body heating by warm shower or bath to improve sleep: A systematic review and meta-analysis", *Sleep Med Rev.*, 46, pp.124–135. DOI: 10.1016/j.smrv.2019.04.008.

9   Eric Suni (16 Dec 2022), "How Smell Affects Your
      Sleep", Sleep Foundation website. Available at: www.
      sleepfoundation.org/bedroom-environment/how-smell-
      affects-your-sleep (Accessed: 17 Feb 2023.)
10   Ibid.
11   NIOSH (n.d.), "Sleep Pressure: Homeostatic Sleep
      Drive", CDC website. Available at: www.cdc.gov/niosh/
      work-hour-training-for-nurses/longhours/mod2/11.html
      (Accessed: 17 Feb 2023.)
12   Danielle Pacheco (7 Feb 2023). "Caffeine and Sleep",
      Sleep Foundation website. Available at: www.
      sleepfoundation.org/nutrition/caffeine-and-sleep

7. Find Your Flow: Intuitive Movement

1   A. Hambleton et al. (2022). "Psychiatric and medical
      comorbidities of eating disorders: findings from a rapid
      review of the literature", *J Eat Disord*, 10, p.132.
2   Zawn Villines (19 Apr 2022). "What a flow state is
      and how to achieve it", MedicalNewsToday website.
      Available at: www.medicalnewstoday.com/articles/
      flow-state (Accessed: 17 Feb 2023.)
3   Seunggu Han (4 Jan 2022). "Dopamine and serotonin:
      Brain chemicals explained", MedicalNewsToday
      website. Available at: www.medicalnewstoday.com/
      articles/326090 (Accessed: 17 Feb 2023.)
4   See T. S. Church et al. (2007). "Effects of Different Doses
      of Physical Activity on Cardiorespiratory Fitness Among
      Sedentary, Overweight or Obese Postmenopausal
      Women With Elevated Blood Pressure: A Randomized
      Controlled Trial", *JAMA*, 297(19), pp.2081–2091.
      DOI:10.1001/jama.297.19.2081
5   ScienceDaily (8 May 2019). "Short bursts of intense
      exercise before meals control blood sugar better
      than 1 continuous 30 minute session", ScienceDaily
      website. Available at: www.sciencedaily.com/
      releases/2014/05/140508192458.htm (Accessed:
      17 Feb 2023.)
6   See Jasmine Bittar (21 Sep 2022). "Alcohol and Fitness",
      Alcohol Rehab Guide website. Available at: www.
      alcoholrehabguide.org/treatment/alcohol-and-fitness/
      (Accessed: 9 Mar 2023.)
7   The Wellness Corner (Dec 2022). "Just 5 Minutes
      of Exercise Can Reduce Your Appetite For Alcohol",
      The Wellness Corner website. Available at: www.

thewellnesscorner.com/blog/5-minutes-of-exercise-as-alcohol-detox. (Accessed: 17 Feb 2023.)

8. Listen to Yourself: Develop Somatic Intuition

1   Cleveland Clinic (n.d.), "Psychosomatic Disorder", Cleveland Clinic website. Available at: my.clevelandclinic.org/health/diseases/21521-psychosomatic-disorder (Accessed: 17 Feb 2023.)

9. Chill Out: Cold Exposure Therapy

1   Eléonore Beurel, Marisa Toups, Charles B. Nemeroff (2020). "The Bidirectional Relationship of Depression and Inflammation: Double Trouble", *Neuron*, 107 (2), pp.234–56. DOI: 10.1016/j.neuron.2020.06.002. Available at: www.sciencedirect.com/science/article/pii/S0896627320304311.

2   Ibid.

3   H. J. Wang, S. Zakhari S and M. K. Jung (21 Mar 2010). "Alcohol, inflammation, and gut-liver-brain interactions in tissue damage and disease development", *World J Gastroenterol*, 16(11), pp.1304–13. DOI: 10.3748/wjg.v16.i11.1304.

4   Institute for Quality and Efficiency in Health Care (IQWiG) (23 Nov 2010). "What is an inflammation?", InformedHealth.org [Internet]. [Updated 2018 Feb 22]. Available from: www.ncbi.nlm.nih.gov/books/NBK279298/ (Accessed 18 Feb 2023.)

5   Innerfire BV (n.d.). "How to deal with depression", Wim Hof Method website. Available at: www.wimhofmethod.com/how-to-deal-with-depression (Accessed: 18 Feb 2023.)

6   Huberman Lab (n.d.). "The Science & Use of Cold Exposure for Health & Performance", *Huberman Lab* (podcast). Available at: hubermanlab.com/the-science-and-use-of-cold-exposure-for-health-and-performance/ (Accessed: 18 Feb 2023.)

7   Ibid.

8   Innerfire BV (n.d.). "Increase your happiness", Wim Hof Method website. Available at: www.wimhofmethod.com/increase-your-happiness (Accessed: 18 Feb 2023.)

9   Ibid.

10   Innerfire BV (n.d.). "Workout recovery", Wim Hof
      Method website. Available at: www.wimhofmethod.
      com/workout-recovery (Accessed: 18 Feb 2023.)
11   Innerfire BV (n.d.). "Lower your blood pressure", Wim
      Hof Method website. Available at: www.wimhofmethod.
      com/lower-your-blood-pressure (Accessed: 18 Feb 2023.)
12   Cleveland Clinic (n.d.), "Metabolism", Cleveland Clinic
      website. Available at: my.clevelandclinic.org/health/
      body/21893-metabolism (Accessed: 18 Feb 2023.)
13   Innerfire BV (n.d.). "Improve your metabolism", Wim
      Hof Method website. Available at: www.wimhofmethod.
      com/improve-your-metabolism (Accessed: 18 Feb 2023.)
14   Rod Brouhard (3 Oct 2022). "How to Avoid Ice Burn
      When Treating an Injury", verywellhealth website.
      Available at: www.verywellhealth.com/frostbite-with-
      an-ice-pack-1298334
15   IPRS Health (10 Oct 2022). "8 Benefits of Cold Water
      Swimming", IPRS Health website. Available at: www.
      iprshealth.com/news/8-benefits-of-cold-water-
      swimming/ (Accessed: 18 Feb 2023.)

10. Turn Inward: Breathwork and Meditation

1   Counseling Center, University of Toledo (n.d.). "Deep
      Breathing and Relaxation", University of Toledo website.
      Available from: www.utoledo.edu/studentaffairs/
      counseling/anxietytoolbox/breathingandrelaxation.html
      (Accessed: 16 Feb 2023.)
2   Karthik Kumar (18 Nov 2021). "Why Do Navy SEALs
      Use Box Breathing?", MedicineNet website. Available at:
      www.medicinenet.com/why_do_navy_seals_use_box_
      breathing/article.htm (Accessed: 16 Feb 2023.)
3   Andrew Weil (n.d.). "Three Breathing Exercises and
      Techniques", Dr Weil website. Available at: www.drweil.
      com/health-wellness/body-mind-spirit/stress-anxiety/
      breathing-three-exercises/ (Accessed: 16 Feb 2023.)
4   See Y. Álvarez-Pérez et al. (13 Mar 2022). "Effectiveness
      of Mantra-Based Meditation on Mental Health: A
      Systematic Review and Meta-Analysis", *Int J Environ
      Res Public Health*, 19(6), p.3380. DOI: 10.3390/
      ijerph19063380.
5   See Cristina Serrano, Yolanda Andreu, and Sergio
      Murgui (2020), "The Big Five and subjective wellbeing:
      The mediating role of optimism", *Psicothema*, 32(3),
      pp.352–8. DOI: 10.7334/psicothema2019.392.

11. Tune In: Sound Healing

1   Author Zoom call with Farzana Ali (10 Oct 2022).
2   BetterHelp Editorial Team (13 Dec 2022). "What are Alpha Brain Waves?", BetterHelp website. Available at: www.betterhelp.com/advice/general/what-are-alpha-brain-waves/ (Accessed: 9 Feb 2023.)
3   See Mayo Clinic Staff (n.d.), "Stress Management", Mayo Clinic website. Available at: www.mayoclinic.org/healthy-lifestyle/stress-management/in-depth/stress-symptoms/art-20050987 (Accessed: 9 Feb 2023.)
4   Private email correspondence with Summer Muse.
5   Eddie Weitzberg and Jon O. N. Lundberg (15 Jul 2002). "Humming Greatly Increases Nasal Nitric Oxide", *Am J Respir Crit Care Med*, 166(2), pp.144–5.

12. Write It Out: Journaling

1   Kaiser Permanente (24 Mar 2022). "Why everyone should keep a journal–7 surprising benefits", Kaiser Permanente website. Available at: healthy.kaiserpermanente.org/health-wellness/healtharticle.7-benefits-of-keeping-a-journal (Accessed: 20 Feb 2023.)
2   See Kori D. Miller (18 Jun 2019). "14 Benefits of Practicing Gratitude (Incl. Journaling)", PositivePsychology.com. Available at: positivepsychology.com/benefits-of-gratitude/ (Accessed: 20 Feb 2023.)
3   Ralph Ryback (3 Oct 2016). "The Science of Accomplishing Your Goals", Psychology Today website. Available at: www.psychologytoday.com/us/blog/the-truisms-wellness/201610/the-science-accomplishing-your-goals (Accessed: 20 Feb 2023.)
4   Danielle Pacheco (31 Jan 2023). "How Do Dreams Affect Sleep?", Sleep Foundation website. Available at: www.sleepfoundation.org/dreams/how-do-dreams-affect-sleep (Accessed: 20 Feb 2023.)
5   Danielle Pacheco (13 Feb 2023). "Deep Sleep: How Much Do You Need?", Sleep Foundation website. Available at: www.sleepfoundation.org/stages-of-sleep/deep-sleep (Accessed: 20 Feb 2023.)

13. Reclaim Your Power: Conscious Manifestation

1   Lara Doherty (1 Nov 2022). "The Science Behind Vision Boards", The Motivation Clinic website. Available at: www.themotivationclinic.co.uk/blog/blog-post-title-three-grwe9 (Accessed: 20 Feb 2023.)

14. Build a Community: Create Your Soberish Support System

1   Sheri Jacobson (4 Jun 2022). "Your 'Shadow' Self – What It Is, And How It Can Help You", Harley Therapy website. Available at: www.harleytherapy.co.uk/counselling/shadow-self.htm (Accessed: 20 Feb 2023.)

15. Beating Backsliding Behaviours

1   GoodTherapy (20 Aug 2018). "Isolation", GoodTherapy website. Available at: www.goodtherapy.org/learn-about-therapy/issues/isolation (Accessed: 20 Feb 2023.)
2   Valencia Higuera (28 Jul 2022). "Situational depression or clinical depression", MedicalNewsToday website. Available at: www.medicalnewstoday.com/articles/314698 (Accessed: 20 Feb 2023.)
3   Matthew Glowiak (14 Apr, 2020). "What is Self-Care and Why is it Important For You?", Southern New Hampshire University website. Available at: www.snhu.edu/about-us/newsroom/health/what-is-self-care (Accessed 21 Feb 2023.)
4   Greater Good Science Center (n.d.). "Gratitude Defined", Greater Good Magazine website. Available at: greatergood.berkeley.edu/topic/gratitude/definition#what-is-gratitude (Accessed: 21 Feb 2023.)
5   Jennifer Weeks (11 Mar 2021). "Emotional Self-Care in 2021", Student Well-being Blog, John Hopkins University website. Available at: wellbeing.jhu.edu/blog/2021/03/11/emotional-self-in-2021/ (Accessed: 21 Feb 2023.)
6   Dylan Walsh (14 Sep 2022). "Study: Social media use linked to decline in mental health", MIT Sloan School of Management website. Available at: mitsloan.mit.edu/ideas-made-to-matter/study-social-media-use-linked-to-decline-mental-health (Accessed: 21 Feb 2023.)

7   World Health Organization (28 May 2019). "Burn-out an 'occupational phenomenon': International Classification of Diseases", WHO website. Available at: www.who. int/news/item/28-05-2019-burn-out-an-occupational-phenomenon-international-classification-of-diseases (Accessed: 21 Feb 2023.)

8   See Dustin A. Pardini, et al. (2000). "Religious faith and spirituality in substance abuse recovery: Determining the mental health benefits", *Journal of Substance Abuse Treatment*, 19(4), pp. 347–54. Available at: www.sciencedirect.com/science/article/pii/S0740547200001252. (Accessed: 7 Mar 2023.)

16. New Me, Who Dis?: Recreating Our Self-Identity

1   Rylan Calderaro (27 Mar 2021). "Reducing Social Anxiety: The Spotlight Effect", The Cabrini Blog webpage. Available at: www.cabrini.edu/blog/2020-2021-blogs/reducing-social-anxiety-the-spotlight-effect (Accessed: 21 Feb 2023.)

2   See C. D. Ryff (2014). "Psychological well-being revisited: advances in the science and practice of Eudaimonia", *Psychother Psychosom*, 83(1), pp10–28. DOI: 10.1159/000353263.

17. Ready, Set, Show Time

1   Andrew Benson (14 Jan 2023). "Alcohol consumption on the decline for Gen Z, studies suggest", Global News website. Available at: globalnews.ca/news/9411516/alcohol-consumption-decline-gen-z/ (Accessed: 22 Feb 2023.)

Acknowledgements

As someone in constant search for larger ways to be of service to the sober and soberish community, I couldn't imagine a better way to spread my message than a book. Lucky for me the universe brought me Lucy. Thank you to Lucy Carroll for commissioning and believing that I was capable of doing something I never even knew I had in me. Thank you to the rockstar Watkins team who made this book possible and beyond what I could have ever imagined – Sue Lascelles, Brittany Willis, Sophie Elletson, Laura Whitaker-Jones, Emily Jarman, Octavia Lavender, Vikki Scott and Gigi St John. I am indebted to you all for your work on making Soberish come to life, I believe it's truly going to help so many people.

To my network of friends and experts, I will be forever grateful for the time taken for your incredible contributions: Nikita Mehta, Marcus Bradley, Emma Mumford, Lindsay Dalton, Dr Brooke Scheller, Dr Jeff Simone, Farzana Ali, Summer Muse, Kiola Raines and Gillian Tietz. And to all of those in the community I interviewed who shared their experiences to help others, thank you for being of service.

Thank you to my family, care team and loved ones for your unconditional love and support. I am privileged to have so many wonderful people in my life who not only forgave my past mistakes, but continued to be an integral part of my healing process throughout my recovery. Without your belief in my capabilities to transform my pain and trauma into something bigger than myself, I genuinely do not believe I would be here today. You loved me, for me, in times I could not love myself.

To my parents, Renee and David, I hope that this book can show you how far I've come, and how Kurt and I are blessed beyond words to have you as our guiding lights. You have raised and shaped two young adults who are doing their best to change the world for the better; our resilience, grit, intelligence, compassion and empathy all have come from you. I am proud to be your daughter and I hope this book brings you the same pride I feel.

About the Author

Kayla Lyons is the founder of Join Soberish and 1,000 Hours Dry (The Dry Club), inclusive online communities dedicated to those looking to change their relationship with alcohol. She is also a founding team member of Reframe App. Kayla has been in recovery from substance abuse since 2016 and is an active advocate for more affordable, accessible treatment and resources. Kayla lives in Newport Beach, California and enjoys spending her free time with her French Bulldog Winston, exploring new restaurants and fitness boutiques with her friends and teaching Lagree pilates classes.